## CREATING A NEW SALT-FREE DIET

When Peter Brunswick, public relations consultant, experienced a high blood pressure "episode," Dr. Assa Weinberg prescribed a low-sodium diet.

Aware that sodium is indeed a "silent killer," Dr. Weinberg reduced Peter's salt intake to a minimum and monitored the results frequently.

Convinced that salt-free living didn't have to mean the end of good eating, Peter's friend Dorothy Love, an award-winning theatrical producer, began researching low-sodium foods and inventing tasty recipes. She soon enlisted Peter's help in creating and preparing new dishes.

The results of their collaboration were twofold: an exciting new salt-free diet and a happy marriage.

# HOW TO LIVE 365 DAYS A YEAR THE SALT-FREE WAY

BY J. PETER BRUNSWICK,
DOROTHY LOVE
AND ASSA WEINBERG, M.D.

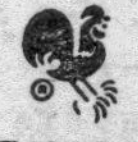

BANTAM BOOKS
TORONTO · NEW YORK · LONDON · SYDNEY

HOW TO LIVE 365 DAYS A YEAR THE SALT-FREE WAY

*A Bantam Book / June 1977*

*2nd printing ............ July 1977*
*3rd printing .. September 1977*
*4th printing .......... March 1978*
*5th printing ...... October 1978*
*6th printing .......... March 1980*
*7th printing ............. July 1981*



ISBN 0-553-20409-2

*Published simultaneously in the United States and Canada*

---



---

PRINTED IN THE UNITED STATES OF AMERICA

16 15 14 13 12 11 10 9 8

# Contents

# Introduction

This is the experience of three people, Peter, his friend Dorothy and a young physician named Assa, and how they dealt with Peter's diet problems when it was discovered that Peter suffered from high blood pressure.

It would be misleading to describe these three or the lives they lead as either ordinary or typical.

Peter is a writer in middle age and of European background, currently public relations counsel to an international airline. To bring his blood pressure under control, a doctor had put him on drugs and had prescribed a low-sodium diet. As Peter tells it, no one, including the physician prescribing it, seemed to know precisely what was involved in such a diet and how to stick to so unpalatable a regimen for any length of time. He was told to "spare the saltshaker and lay off regular bread and salty soups." He followed those vague instructions as best he could, but the result was less than encouraging. At that point he met and became friends with Assa, a young internist and told him his story. When they went over Peter's diet together, Assa concluded that sodium was the culprit. He read everything he could lay his hands on that dealt with the effects of sodium on the human body; studies that had been done as far back as fifty years ago. He became convinced that sodium was indeed a "Silent Killer." Assa is a cross between a Ralph Nader-type medical crusader and an angry-young-man-type physician who cares as deeply about preventive medicine as he does about curing the ill. He reduced Peter's daily sodium intake to a minimum and monitored the results frequently.

The invaluable third partner to this team effort was Dorothy. She is a strikingly attractive woman who has spent most of her life in the musical theater, first as a dancer, singer and actress and later as a theater owner and producer of an award-winning musical. She has combined a career in show business with that of mother and housewife, without so much as a passing glance at the Women's Lib movement. A shrewd business woman with a warm, exceedingly feminine personality, she was widowed and left to bring up two small daughters. She and Peter, who had been divorced some years ago, had fallen in love instantly when a friend introduced them and they decided to build a new life together. She is given much of the credit for the success of the low-sodium regimen devised by Assa and followed by Peter to this day.

Their story is an inspiring example of how medical energy, combined with love and resourcefulness, can turn a troublesome affliction into an exciting adventure in living.

*The Editor*

# The Doctor Speaks

# 1

# The Silent Killer

Dear Reader:

The point of this book is simple and straightforward. It needs no fifteen-letter medical words. Here it is. In the last 20 years of scientific research, it has become increasingly clear that salt, the table condiment, in the quantities we use every day is toxic and a slow-acting poison. Its continuous use leads to or helps in the development of a disease called high blood pressure.

Let me be very blunt. High blood pressure is a mortal disease. It kills. It kills many people every year. It's not only fatal but extremely common. The facts are that one out of 10 Americans suffers from this disease. This means that more than 20 million people in this country, whites, blacks, men, women, people from all walks of life—have high blood pressure. Twenty million people is a huge number—equivalent to the combined populations of Belgium and The Netherlands, and more than the combined population of two of the world's largest metropolises, New York and Tokyo.

Because of the extent of the disease, hypertension, the term used by doctors to designate high blood pressure, has become a major area of investigation and research. Multiple studies demonstrate that a simple low-salt diet, without any additional drugs, can be an effective therapy for this disease. Five to seven million out of the 20 million Americans affected can control their hypertension just by reducing their salt intake.

In other words, if every hypertensive American were to maintain a low-salt diet, one out of four would be able to control his blood pressure.

Recent research is even more suggestive. Not only can limited salt intake *control* hypertension, but scientists and high blood pressure specialists are now becoming convinced that it is the regular use of the saltshaker that *causes* the disease. Evidence for this is direct in experimental animals and the evidence for humans, though indirect, is substantial.

The human appetite for salt has far surpassed its need. The amount of salt we consume is almost totally governed by culture, customs and food habits acquired very early in life. We have all become salt addicts. No other animal in the world eats as much salt as man. The time has clearly come for us to change our salt habits. Preventive medicine is better than a cure.

This is not a book meant for patients only. It addresses everyone, especially every American mother and father, those who feed the next generation. We now know that our salt habit is dangerous and that there is something we can do about it. Something all of us can do—whether we're a patient or a nonpatient, a private citizen or a public official, a food manufacturer or a consumer. It was to inform all of us about what we can do to prevent the next generation from having so many millions of hypertensives, in hospital beds or in outpatient clinics, that this book is written.

## I. On the track of the silent killer

At the beginning of the 20th century a team of Harvard scientists discovered that animals did not grow in the absence of sodium chloride—a crystal more commonly known as table salt. A certain amount of salt, it seemed, is necessary to maintain life.

It took more than fifty years of research to realize that the opposite is also true: *Excessive* salt intake leads to the development of a mortal disease, hypertension, the third major cause of death in this country.

This discovery was chiefly the work of Walter Kempner, Professor of Medicine at Duke University, and Lewis K. Dahl, Senior Scientist at Brookhaven National Laboratories and the Atomic Energy Commission.

The evidence for the toxic effect of salt came from two sources, animal experimentation and research on humans. Usually scientific truths are first discovered through experiments on animals. Only after sufficient knowledge is gained to minimize the risk does human experimentation begin. This was not the case with salt.

In 1904, two French scientists, Ambard and Beaujard, published a paper in one of the best French medical journals of that time. The subject of the article was a new diet, low in salt, and its effectiveness in reducing high blood pressure. The paper was too short and it contained little scientific data. This may be the reason it did not attract public attention; its thesis was completely ignored for the next 16 years.

In 1920, a textbook on the treatment of kidney disease by F. M. Allen, a renal specialist, appeared in the United States. This time a considerable amount of scientific data showed the efficacy of a low-sodium regimen in the treatment of high blood pressure. But again, nobody attached much importance to this discovery.

Over the next 24 years the idea of a low-salt diet was completely forgotten, and patients with this chronic disease were condemned to an early death, in the same way as patients with tuberculosis were before the discovery of antibiotics.

A year before the end of World War II, Walter Kempner presented the results of a new treatment before the section on the Practice of Medicine of the Medical Society of the state of North Carolina. The new treatment was a diet. It consisted of rice, fruit juice, vitamins and iron. According to Kempner, the diet was able to halt progressive destruction of the heart, kidneys and eyes—the three targets of the hypertension disease. During the previous four years, he had treated 140 high blood pressure patients with the diet, many in a very advanced stage. On May 3,

1944, Kempner showed the results: elevated pressure became markedly reduced, enlarged hearts returned to their normal size, deteriorated kidneys regained normal function. The dangerous process in the eyes that usually leads to complete blindness was entirely arrested. Damaged retinas healed, and patients who had been blind regained their eyesight. In no instance was the diet proven to be harmful.

Kempner's diet attracted worldwide attention. Everywhere physicians urged their hypertensive patients to switch to the rice diet. But a number of unpleasant aspects to Kempner's diet prevented it from being widely adopted. The diet was monotonous and it did not taste good; medicine of this kind is never very agreeable. One had to adhere to the diet for quite awhile before its effect became apparent. Lengthy hospitalization was required until blood pressure was controlled; multiple urine and blood tests had to be taken repeatedly. Many patients tried to modify the diet slightly to suit their tastes, but even minimal additions made the diet worthless. As many said at the time, the rice diet tasted awful and the only excuse for its existence was that it worked.

Nobody knew why, not even Kempner himself. Certain doctors suggested that the curative effect of the rice was due to its high content of vegetable protein. Others thought it was the low cholesterol values. There was even a suggestion that rice might contain a natural substance that could cure high blood pressure.

It took more than a year of intensive laboratory work to solve the mystery of Kempner's diet. The answer was salt. The rice diet was extremely low in sodium—the chemical element that gives the salty taste. Not rice, but the absence of salt in rice brought about the amazing results. Hence, any diet very low in sodium could achieve the same effects. This was an old idea. It was the same theory Ambard and Beaujard had advanced some 40 years before.

Between 1945 and 1960, low-salt diets replaced the monotonous rice diet as a treatment for hypertension. Many patients, including those with severe cases of hypertension, patients who had previously required several medications every day, now found they were able to control their disease by diet alone. No more expensive medicine, only food—and delicious food at that! In later chapters, Peter and Dorothy will tell what a low-salt diet is and how to prepare rich, tasty meals that are low in salt.

Just how many patients with high blood pressure can control their condition with such a diet? In an extensive study done over a period of 25 years at the National Laboratories in Brookhaven, New York, it was found that 25%–33% of all hypertensive patients could be successfully treated by diet alone. The rest were better controlled by a combination of diet and drugs. As a matter of fact, the severity and duration of the symptoms, as well as survival times were much better in the group treated with a combination of diet and drugs than in the group that used drugs alone. These results have been confirmed by many other studies. Since then low-sodium diets have become basic to the treatment of high blood pressure in the United States.

The implication seems clear enough: If you have high blood pressure you should adhere to a low-salt diet, but too many people do not know this—too many, a few million!

This enormous group consists of those who do not want to know and those who do not know. The first are patients who know they have high blood pressure, are under the care of a physician and take their daily medications. They tried the diet once, improperly, failed and never want to hear about it again. They are erroneously convinced that they cannot do without salt. Chapter 3 of this book will deal exclusively with the psychological, physiological and practical problems of our salty taste. There is no basis for the common belief that we cannot enjoy low-salt foods. It's not only wrong to think so, but dangerous.

The second group consists of people who have never heard about a low-salt diet because they do not even know they have high blood pressure! Their number—

four million people. Hard to believe, isn't it? How do we know this? Multiple national surveys done by the Bureau of Health Statistics of the National Institute of Health indicate that one out of 10 people surveyed had high blood pressure. For a country with a population above 200 million this means that more than 20 million Americans living right now have this disease.

The same studies found two frightening facts that should be of national concern, if not cause for public scandal: Twenty percent of the total hypertensives surveyed did not know they had high blood pressure. This is how the four million figure was obtained. Secondly, only 31.8% of known hypertensives were under medical care. In other words, 14 million out of the 20 million people who have high blood pressure are not receiving medical care.

The reason for this outrageous situation? Most Americans believe high blood pressure to be a benign, painless disease, apparently easy to live with. But only apparently! In reality hypertension is a cruel mortal disease, the third leading cause of death in this country. It is the major cause of strokes—a condition that comes upon its victims quite suddenly and not only leaves half the body paralyzed, but in many cases destroys the ability to speak or to understand the spoken word. It is among the major causes of blindness. High blood pressure contributes heavily to the need for artificial kidney and renal transplantation.

## II. Recommendations for reaching and treating hypertensives

There is no escape from the ugly reality of the American high blood pressure. Millions do not care, four million do not even know.

We must reach these millions; this includes people of all ages, especially young adults and the parents of small children. We must inform them. We must tell them that everyone who has high blood pressure and continues to eat salty foods runs the risk of becoming paralyzed, speechless or blind. Every medical student knows it. Every first-year resident in a hospital sees it. To suffer a stroke at the age of 40 that could have been prevented is one of the biggest punishments anyone could inflict on himself. And it happens. Uncontrolled high blood pressure does not give warning —it just strikes!

There are solutions to this problem of reaching and treating hypertensives. These solutions require action on two different scales, national and individual. Much has been done on the national level; the American Heart Association carries on this work every day of the year. But we think this is not enough. We believe additional measures are required and our suggestions for action on the national level are included in Section X.

Of course, a major part of the solution lies with us. We need not wait for the President or an act of Congress. There are practical, down-to-earth, responsible actions that we can and must take now.

- Have your blood pressure checked at regular intervals.
- Have your family's blood pressure checked.
- If one of your household is hypertensive, replace salt with a salt substitute.
- If you are involved in community action, diffuse this information about preventing and controlling hypertension.

The average hypertensive patient remains in bed 8.8 days every year as a direct result of his disease. More than 9.5 million working days are lost annually because of high blood pressure. This number is far smaller than the actual number because it reflects only the employed hypertensives who report in sick. It does not take into account the totally disabled or the very ill patients who are permanently out of work. It does not reflect the hypertensives who are self-employed and do not report their sick days.

High blood pressure is an expensive disease. Medication, when prescribed, should be taken daily and the costs vary from 30¢ a day to more than $1, according to the severity of the disease. This alone means an annual expenditure of between $100 and $500. Strict adherence to a low-salt diet helps to reduce the cost of the disease to patients substantially in both financial and bodily terms.

A public information and action campaign is of particular importance in the black community. The number of unrecognized cases is greater and the number of those under care is smaller than among whites: The salt content of black American meals is high and this is a significant factor in the severity of hypertension among blacks. High blood pressure is uncommon in Africa but is found to be high among Egyptians who eat salty food.

It is encouraging that science has discovered a diet that can control high blood pressure; that five to seven million hypertensives can be treated by diet alone, if only they knew it.

Our task is to let them know.

## III. The salt diet: preventive as well as cure

By 1946 we had evidence that reduced salt consumption could arrest the fatal course of high blood pressure. But we still knew very little about what *caused* the disease, by what mechanism it operated and how it could be prevented from occurring.

The most striking fact was our ignorance, and the discovery of the low-salt diet as an effective treatment only raised more questions. Why and in what way does a low-salt diet cure high blood pressure? What are the long-term effects of a low-salt diet? What is the maximum amount of salt a diet should contain? And perhaps most important: If low salt consumption can cure high blood pressure, can it prevent the disease from ever occurring?

Unfortunately for the medical researchers, no other animal besides man develops high blood pressure. The absence of animal models was a serious handicap to research. New ideas, new drugs cannot be tested directly on human patients, not without prior experimentation on animals. The fact that spontaneous high blood pressure was an exclusively human disease led many people to believe that hypertension was a condition of civilization, caused by pollution, noise and the permanent rush of modern life.

Soon, however, researchers in the field found they were able to induce hypertension in experimental animals—first by surgery and later by introducing large amounts of salt into their diet.

By 1953 there was evidence that, if fed a lot of salt, mice, kangaroo rats, albino rats, rabbits, dogs and cows all developed high blood pressure. Salt did not seem to be the harmless tasty substance we had thought. On the contrary, there was a growing body of proof that salt is a toxic substance, at least in animals. Were we humans also acting as guinea pigs by eating so much salt?

The first frightening evidence was produced by George R. Meneely, an investigator from Vanderbilt University. He started to feed laboratory rats with salty food on a daily basis. Many developed high blood pressure and died after 17 months. The normal life span of this animal is 24 to 48 months. The autopsy proved that their kidneys were damaged, their hearts enlarged—just as in humans with high blood pressure. Even their cause of death—strokes, heart attacks and pneumonia—was frighteningly similar to hypertensive humans. The most convincing fact was that high blood pressure appeared in the animals after nine months on the salty diet. This period corresponds to the beginning of the animal's middle age—the most prevalent period in which high blood pressure develops in man.

This mirror image between animals and humans was too accurate to be considered just coincidental. Perhaps most frightening was that the quantity of salt added to the animal food was equivalent to the daily content of salt in the average American diet!

The next 20 years of research into the connection between high blood pressure and salt were dominated by the same Lewis K. Dahl whose name we mentioned earlier. Since 1954 his work at the Brookhaven National Laboratories has been dedicated to understanding the effects of regular table salt on the human body. At the time Dahl began his investigative work, knowledge of the biological effects of salt could be contained in a few typed papers. Today I had to use a computer to obtain all the known data.

Like many others, Dahl was perplexed by the Meneely experiments. The fact that the normal salt content of American meals could induce high blood pressure in animals was highly provocative. But what attracted Dahl's attention was that not *all* the animals that consumed salty food developed high blood pressure; a few of the Meneely rats remained healthy for the rest of their normal life span of two to four years.

Dahl began his work by feeding a new group of rats with salty nutrition, equivalent to the average American meals. Their blood pressure was taken at regular intervals. After the first nine months of the salty diet, many of the rats became hypertensive, but many did not. Dahl then chose the male and the female with the highest blood pressure in the group and placed them in a new cage so they could mate. This couple had six offspring and the whole family was fed with salty food. A second year passed. At the end of this period, the blood pressure of the offspring was checked. This time the *majority* of the new generation had high blood pressure and only a few did not. Again Dahl selected the male and the female with the highest pressure, mated them in a new cage and the third generation feeding began.

This type of experiment is long and difficult. It takes almost a year to develop high blood pressure in an animal by daily salt feeding. In the meantime animals can die from infections or other causes. If too many animals die, the experiment has to start again from the first generation. Another year passed. When the third generation matured, the picture became clear. *All* the members of this generation were hypertensive.

From Dahl's work we learned that high blood pressure is transmissible. High blood pressure is a genetic disease. Many of us carry inside our cells a genetic bomb, inherited from our parents, which explodes—manifests itself—only in our middle age. This explains why a few of the experimental animals survived despite constant salt feeding. They were born without this special gene.

The discovery that hypertension was a genetic disease was certainly important, but it did not answer the major question: Can a low-salt diet prevent the appearance of high blood pressure in an animal carrying the gene? To answer this question, Dahl used the animals of the fourth generation. All the members of this generation inherited the defective gene from their parents. These animals were destined to develop high blood pressure in their adult life and to die prematurely. But from birth, Dahl gave them a low-salt diet exclusively. None of the animals developed high blood pressure, despite their genetic inheritance.

This was indisputable evidence that a low-salt diet can prevent the appearance of the fatal disease, high blood pressure, and it created a real stir in preventive medicine circles. For the first time a real fear spread among nutritionists and epidemiologists about the salt habits of our society. Especially the salt content in the food of babies and young children. This was in 1962.

Since then, it has been demonstrated many times that:

The younger the age at which salt is first consumed, the earlier high blood pressure appears!

The longer period of time salt is consumed, the more severe the hypertension will be!

The richer the diet is in salt, the younger the animal will die!

One fact should be reiterated: The quantity of salt used in all of these experiments is equivalent to 30–240 grains a day—the *daily* content of the *normal* American diet!

## IV. How much salt is safe for humans?

Can salted food *cause* high blood pressure in humans? This question troubled many nations in the Western world where salt is a major additive and high blood pressure a major cause of death. The answer could be found only among civilizations which do not use salt. In most cases, ironically, these were the primitive societies.

In 1951, Dahl called the American Museum of Natural History in New York to find out about the use of salt among primitive tribes, a question no one had explored before. He finally spoke with someone who had just come back from visiting a remote tribe in South America. High blood pressure among members of this tribe was nonexistent. "Do they use salt?" asked Dahl. "Oh my, yes, they all carried it around in small bags," answered the scientist. "It is used for money, never on food, you know."

Anthropologists knew of at least five human groups that had never tasted salt other than what their natural diet contained. These were Eskimos near the North Pole, a certain part of the Kikuyu tribe in Kenya, fighters of the Masai tribe in East Africa, most Northwestern American Indians and certain Chinese. The urine of these groups contained less than 16 grains of salt per day (30–240 grains in the United States). They found their food in nature, but not all followed vegetarian diets.

The Eskimos, in fact, are the most carnivorous eaters among the human race. An average Eskimo consumes 6,000 calories in 24 hours. This is three times the intake of the average American: 4,500 calories or 4½ pounds (2 kilograms) come from animal meat and not less than 1,500 calories are fat. In spite of the considerable amount of meat and fat, high blood pressure and heart attacks are rare among Eskimos. The only sodium in their diet comes from what is naturally in their food. Four and one-half pounds of animal meat contain 25 grains of salt: this is six times less than most Americans consume.

The diet of the Masai tribe in Africa consists of meat, milk and blood. High blood pressure is virtually nonexistent, and their urine contains only 16 grains of sodium a day.

High blood pressure was not found among certain Indians from South Bolivia and islanders from Samoa and Hawaii and, accordingly, it was found that they did not use salt.

This was further indirect confirmation of Dahl's theory: That the nonuse of table salt in food prevents the appearance of high blood pressure. The first real corroboration of the toxic effect of salt as an additive in modern society came from Japan. In the years that followed World War II, the standard of living of most Japanese increased markedly. Death from contagious diseases like tuberculosis decreased, and cancer and vascular diseases became the major cause of mortality, just as in the Western world. But, unlike Americans, Japanese did not die of heart attacks. Arteriosclerosis was found to be a rare phenomenon in Japan. The main cause of death was cerebral hemorrhage, induced by high blood pressure.

In the Atica Province in northern Japan, there were twice as many deaths from high blood pressure than in Okayama in the south. The incidence of hypertension above the age of 50 in the north was inexplicably high—two out of three people—the highest incidence in the world. In the south only one out of 10 people had high blood pressure. Many attempts to identify the cause of the high mortality in the north failed. The diet of both populations was studied in detail, but no difference was found in calorie, protein, calcium or vitamin intake. There was only one significant difference—salt.

Dr. Fuduka from Shiba University measured the salt of the northern Japanese diet. It contained almost an ounce (0.88 ounces) of salt daily. It was much less in the south (0.59 ounces). Both north and south consumed the same vegetables, pickles, soy sauce and other foodstuffs. The different item was the *miso*, the famous Japanese soup. It contained 90 *grains* more salt in the north than in the south. The salt content of the *miso* soup in the north was solely responsible for the increased mortality from high blood pressure. But the most striking demonstration of the poisonous effect of long-term use of salt was the discovery of a primitive society that uses salt.

In 1968, British investigators discovered an island in Polynesia where the population used salt. On a neighboring island they did not. On these two islands Dahl's theory was confirmed in full. There were many hypertensives on the island of salt users but almost none on the other.

A few studies that tried to relate high blood pressure and salt could not confirm the relationship. A study of natives of New Guinea found similar blood pressure in groups with different salt intake. A study among black West Indians found the same salt consumption among people with high blood pressure as among people with normal pressure. A study in Cleveland found that a family history of hypertension has a greater influence on the development of the disease than excessive salt intake. But this study did find that the severity of the disease was affected by excessive salt intake. I do not intend to underestimate the importance of these studies. But their effect is not to invalidate every other study. They merely indicate that salt is not the only factor, unfortunately, in causing hypertension. What other factors contribute to the disease remain to be discovered. But there is still conclusive evidence of the dangerous association between the use of salt as a food additive and the incidence of high blood pressure.

## V. Obesity and high blood pressure: exploding some myths

At least one reason for the large number of undiagnosed hypertensives is the public conviction that hypertension is a disease of the obese.

It is a popular belief in our society that overweight is the cause of high blood pressure. Many weight reduction programs claim that a fall in blood pressure will follow the adoption of a low-calorie diet, and this has led many hypertensive people to join such programs. Unfortunately, there is very little scientific evidence to support these claims.

In fact, investigators have found that accumulated fat has little or no influence on blood pressure. However, excessive eating of regular American foodstuffs leads inevitably to more salt consumption; hence it is the high salt intake, not the rich diet, that accounts for the incidence of high blood pressure among the obese. Again it was Lewis Dahl who discovered this fascinating fact. Dahl conducted a series of experiments in 1958 on overweight, hypertensive patients to measure the value of a low-salt diet versus a weight reduction program in controlling high blood pressure. Dahl divided his patients into three groups. The first used regular amounts of salt, but followed a very severe low-calorie regimen. Weight loss in this group was a success—17 to 57 pounds (8–26 kilograms) per patient in a few months—but there was not even a single case of reduction in blood pressure.

The second group of obese hypertensive patients was treated with a very rich, high-calorie diet that contained a very low amount of sodium. The unexpected happened: The majority of this group had a significant improvement in their blood pressure, in spite of the absence of weight loss. In order to reduce blood pressure by weight loss alone, it was necessary that the third group lose not only all excess fat, but an additional 20% from the weight considered ideal.

There is no question that obesity does lead to many serious health problems: heart attacks, sudden death, deterioration of joint surface and a shorter life span. These known complications of overweight *can* be prevented by low-calorie diets. But low-calorie diets *cannot* prevent high blood pressure, just as low-salt diets cannot prevent the complications of obesity.

There may be yet another explanation for the false impression among the public that high blood pressure is a disease of the obese. The blood pressure apparatus used by many American physicians is too short (14 inches or 26 centimeters); it cannot completely encircle the arms of 70% of the adult population of the United States! It has been known since 1900 that too short a cuff produces a mistake in the machine reading, which may lead to a wrong diagnosis of hypertension in normal people. A few years ago in Finland, a short-cuff machine caused the impression of a hypertension epidemic among the people examined. The epidemic was "cured" by simply replacing the machine.

Medical authorities in this country should do the same. They should recommend the withdrawal of the short-cuff apparatus and its replacement by the longer-cuff machine already in use by many physicians.

### VI. How salt affects blood pressure

The way salt affects our body remains a mystery, in spite of many attempts to solve it. It has been known since the middle of the nineteenth century that excessive salt consumption activates the thirst mechanism and forces us to drink more water. Drinking water relieves our thirst, but loads the body with an additional volume of fluid that can adversely affect the pressure of the blood. Every pregnant woman knows that eating salt during pregnancy can endanger her life and her baby by causing toxemia, which is nothing but a special form of high blood pressure.

The first theory to gain favor postulated that high blood pressure was caused by salt retention. This was found to be untrue. Studies with radioactive salt showed that people with hypertension do not retain more salt than people without hypertension. After a meal of salty food, the body of a healthy person and of a hypertensive person will retain the same quantity of salt it requires for its maintenance and will slough off any excess. It is, therefore, not the retention of salt, but what salt does to the body while it is there that causes the high blood pressure. How? By slowly damaging the kidneys.

Research over the last 30 years has found that the kidneys play a major role in regulating blood pressure. A substance secreted by this organ into the bloodstream in minute amounts controls the complicated process that builds the pressure in the blood, at least in part. Certain doctors claim that the presence of excessive salt in the body interferes with this vital secretion, deregulates the control mechanism and causes a rise in blood pressure.

It is a regrettable fact that the daily salt intake of the average American exceeds by five to 15 times, and in many cases much more, the quantity he needs to maintain his body in good health. This results in a permanent bombardment of our organism by salt grains, more correctly—sodium, which forces the kidneys, the main blood filter, to remain in constant activity, trying to flush out the huge amount of unnecessary salt. In fact, it takes 24 to 48 hours to filter out normal quantities of salt and five to 10 days if the load is too heavy.

Though we now have some clues into the hypertension mystery, many questions remain unanswered. It is not quite clear, for instance, by what mechanism normal blood pressure is regulated and how the deregulation process takes place. The influence of genetic and environmental factors on the secretion of the control factor is poorly understood. Only further research can bring a complete answer to the problem of salt toxicity.

### VII. How the salt habit is ingrained in children

The first years of life are critical to our mental and physical development. Many of the habits, tastes and values of our adult life are acquired during this period. The salt addiction of Western culture, with its alarming implication for high blood pressure, is one of them. How do we instill a need for salt in our children? By adding salt to our children's food! Why? So that the food will taste better to the adult who buys or cooks it.

It is unbelievable but true. Commercial baby foods from four leading U.S. companies were given to seven laboratory animals from birth as the sole source of nutrition. Four months later, five out of the seven had high blood pressure! A second group of animals fed with the very same baby foods, from which only the salt was extracted, remained normal and did not develop the disease.

Though the need for salt in human infants is greater than in adults, due to the growing process, the need can be met by one-fifth to one-half grain of salt a day (22 = 42mg) during the first weeks of life. Unfortunately, by the end of the first year of life, the quantity of salt normally given to American babies in their food is often as much as twice the amount needed to maintain health.

There is a simple reason for this sad reality. The two major sources of babies' nutrition in the United States—commercial baby food and cow's milk—are flooded with salt. According to "Handbook Number 8" of the Department of Agriculture on the composition of processed food, it appears that:

• Processed meat has 5 to 6 times more salt than it naturally contains.

• Processed vegetables have 6 to 60 times more salt than they naturally contain.

• Cereal contains 100 times more.

Cow's milk is no different. Children have an amazing capacity to adapt to whatever feeding program they are given, but more and more questions are being raised about the long-term undesirable consequences of substituting cow's milk for breast milk. In comparison to human milk, cow's milk contains 50% less digestible protein and 600% more salt. Is it only a coincidence that death from vascular diseases has also increased since the beginning of the century by 600%?

Maternal milk contains a low amount of salt, regardless of how much salt the mother eats. There is no escaping the conclusion that this natural protection against high blood pressure was sacrificed when cow's milk replaced breast feeding as the primary source of infant nutrition at the beginning of this century.

## VIII. How much salt do we really need?

The amount of salt our body needs to maintain itself in good health is amazingly small. As in the case of other minerals, our organism requires a constant salt level and hence losses must be replaced continually.

Salt leaves the body in two major ways: through the urine and the skin. A minor amount is lost along with hair, nails, saliva, stools, etc. The loss varies from day to day but rises substantially whenever climatic conditions force into action the cooling activity of the sweat glands in the skin.

These millions of microscopic glands are capable of pumping out most of the body's salt in a few hours, a process which may even lead to death if the lost salt is not replaced. For this reason, athletes, heavy construction workers and inhabitants of the desert—all those living under conditions that lead to excessive sweating—are required to add salt to their food. But the majority of Americans do not live under such conditions.

The United States is located in the temperate zone, in a climate that does not activate our sweat glands excessively. Therefore, our major loss in salt is through our urine, not our skin. Many studies of the urine of normal and hypertensive volunteers clearly show that the amount of salt excreted in the urine becomes smaller and smaller if the content of this mineral in the diet is progressively reduced. The smaller the salt content of the food, the smaller the salt waste is.

However, when the diet is completely free from salt, the urine still contains a certain amount, which means there is no way to avoid at least some waste. In fact, in the complete absence of salt, the body breaks down its own tissues and utilizes the salt that was used to build the organs in order to maintain this level of waste. (Obviously, such conditions will eventually lead to death.) It is this daily amount of loss that represents our real minimal need for salt.

In other words, in a temperate climate, in the absence of excessive sweating a normal healthy American requires *10 grains of salt a day*, and this quantity should be provided by his diet.

This does not mean that we must use the saltshaker. On the contrary. Salt is a natural constituent of almost every food in nature, both vegetables and meats. The truth is that a regular American diet with no addition of table salt already contains 20 to 60 grains more than the amount necessary to maintain life!

There is clearly no need or advantage to using saltshakers. We strongly urge the American public to abandon this practice that has become so much a part of our way of life.

Can we really do it? Can we lose our taste, our seeming need, for additional salt?

## IX. Are we born salt addicts?

No other creature in the animal world consumes as much salt as man does. The fact that a few animals are known to lick salt led scientists to believe for a period that our taste for salt was genetically determined. This argument is often mistakenly used against reduction of salt in the diet. However, this theory was invalidated many years ago. Salt-licking animals, it was discovered, reside in areas where the salt content of plants, soil and rain is so small that their survival becomes impossible unless an additional source of salt can be found. The salt-licking habit disappears when these animals are transferred to a different region where the natural salt conditions are more favorable. Man is the only animal who salts his food more than his health requirements dictate, and even for him it is a new habit.

We are a 20-million-year-old animal, but salt was discovered by the human race only six thousand years ago. If the span of human existence is compared to a period of 24 hours, the period in which we have used salt occupies only the last 26 seconds. The oldest among human languages, Sanskrit, does not even contain a term for salt, and it is impossible to trace the word among the European languages farther back than the primitive Greek. During most of its known history, salt was a rare and expensive product. In the Roman period, it was used as money, and that is where the word "salary" has its origin. It was only three centuries ago that salt came into popular use. After a thousand years of political battles it was finally made a tax-free product. (Was this an historical mistake?)

Low-salt diets were the life-style of millions of people through many centuries. There is no basis, therefore, to the popular belief that our desire for salt was genetically determined millions of years ago or that a more moderate use runs counter to our nature.

But the salt taste is one of the fundamental pleasures in our present food culture. Does a program that threatens to remove a staple from the diet of 200 million people stand any chance of success? I sincerely believe it does.

I do not fool myself. As a doctor, I have learned not to overestimate the power of medical information to alter living habits. We all know the limited results of the campaigns against alcohol and cigarette smoking. My belief in the future success of the low-salt diet is based on the fact that hundreds of thousands of people in this country are *already* free of saltshakers and still enjoy their food. Hundreds of thousands of people with high blood pressure, who presumably doubted that they could do it—people like you and me. A low-salt culture is, therefore, not just a dream of the future but already part of our present reality.

The threat to a widespread low-salt culture is in the public belief that unsalty food is tasteless. In Western society, where food is a basic pleasure, such a belief guarantees a vigorous resistance to change. But it happens to be untrue. Extensive experience in the last 20 years has proven that we begin to enjoy low-salt food after an adaptation period of two to eight weeks. This does not mean that we resign ourselves to a bland but necessary regimen; it means that we actually discover new sensitivities and tastes that could not be felt before as Peter and Dorothy will show you in the following pages. The low-salt meal does not lose any of its psychological pleasure value, and the consumer continues to find intense satisfaction in food.

Peter agrees that during the adaptation period the unsalted food often tastes bad to most people, but with Dorothy's help, he was able to get through this short period without major difficulty. A minor withdrawal syndrome appears in about 25% of those on the diet during the first week and disappears by itself on the tenth day. It consists of nervousness, fatigue, mild depression and malaise. More intense, but similar phenomena, are seen during withdrawal from other addictions such as alcohol and cigarettes. The existence of a withdrawal syndrome—the fact that the body can develop an unhealthy dependence on sodium—is one of the strongest arguments against the excessive use of salt.

Experience with the effects of long-term low-salt diets is extensively longer than with contraceptive pills, for example. No physical or mental side effects have been known to develop. On the contrary, an unexpected psychological benefit was discovered among long-term users of this diet. Psychological projective tests revealed that one out of four subjects find the world a more pleasant place to live in than they did before adopting a low-salt diet. This surprising result is expressed in better relations with family members and relatives; even department store clerks seem less irritable.

From the practical point of view living on low-salt diets has become easier in the last 10 years. The food industry has responded to the discoverey of the toxic effects of sodium and low-salt products are now on the shelves of many supermarkets and food stores, which makes it possible to satisfy gourmet tastes and still adhere to the diet.

In addition, there are two important reasons why I feel optimistic about the relative success of a fight against the American salt habit.

The health risks of high salt consumption and the price of avoiding them are different than in the case of nicotine and alcohol.

First, the chances of having high blood pressure are many times greater than the chances of contracting lung cancer from cigarettes or cirrhosis of the liver from alcohol. You can draw up your own statistics. Count how many people you know personally that have these diseases and compare this number with the people you know that have high blood pressure. There is no need for a national survey to realize that the chances of avoiding high blood pressure are many times smaller than the chances of avoiding lung cancer or liver disease.

Secondly, I believe that public resistance to an attack on a common pleasure is based not only on a lack of information or the lack of fear, but on the failure to provide an equivalent pleasure substitute that contains no medical risks. Nothing has replaced cigarettes or alcohol. But this is not the case with salt. Low-salt diets, such as this book offers and salt substitutes have proven to be effective salt replacements, thus making the loss acceptable.

The problem in the case of the fight against our salt habit is not the absence of valid substitutes, but the lack of public information on the risks of salt. I am convinced that if the public knew how high the risk and how low the price, most of us would abandon the use of saltshakers.

During the preparation of this book, I had the chance to talk on this subject with people in the black community, with young mothers and others who do not have high blood pressure, and I was amazed to find out the extent and impact of the message this book contains. It encourages me further to believe that if we engage ourselves in an extensive educational campaign, we as well as the next generation will stand a better chance against the many perils of high blood pressure.

Here's what I propose.

## X. An appeal to the American public

Prevention of death and disease has always been one of the noble dreams of mankind and the ultimate goal of medicine. But until now, we have been largely confined to curing those already sick, to repairing what is already damaged. Still impelled by our vision and curiosity, we have never completely abandoned the old dream and today our society has a chance to satisfy part of this ancient goal.

In the last decades many enemies of the public health have been exposed: radiation, alcohol, nicotine and industrial chemicals are but a few. The public took effective measures to protect itself against their danger. We should bring to bear the same spirit in a fight against the toxic effects of salt.

Public protection against salt involves an attack on two ingrained habits: the neglect in disease detection and the use of saltshakers. In the first case, I suggest that American industry take upon itself the development of a machine that can be used by the public to detect high blood pressure. This project is certainly easier and less expensive than many other scientific tasks this country has set for itself. Such machines should be placed in public areas like subways and theaters, in the way scales to measure weight are. There is no reason why the measurement of blood pressure should not become a public habit in the way weight watching has. This could go a long way to helping solve the gigantic problem of undiagnosed hypertension.

The fight against the use of saltshakers should take place everywhere food is served, both in public and at home. Low-salt cooking and salt substitutes should become an available choice in restaurants, hotels, airplanes, etc. Today, despite the 20 million hypertensives among us, this choice is available almost only at hospitals.

A more difficult task is changing our cooking style. Cooking schools and home economics courses should include low-salt recipes in their programs. The addition of salt to food should be reduced gradually at home.

These are the simple but essential acts of modern preventive medicine. Unfortunately, they are largely unknown to the future candidates for high blood pressure—the healthy public. Unless preventive medicine can reach us all, its knowledge is a virtual waste.

To achieve an effective level of public protection against excessive use of salt, I suggest that the three following measures be taken on the national level by Congress and the President.

1) Congress should pass a federal law that will oblige every food manufacturer to print on the label the quantity of salt in grains and grams that its product contains. This will provide every consumer with a choice he does not have now. The impact of a consumer's choice of the brand low in salt will lead to a reduction in the quantity of salt commercially added to all food products.

2) Even more important, Congress should pass a law that will oblige elementary schools and high schools to include preventive medicine in their educational programs. Basic medical information in modern society cannot be disseminated by family physicians alone. The quantity of essential information about how to prevent diseases increases from year to year, while elementary health measures remain unknown to the public. Preventive medicine in schools can build in our children healthy habits and new attitudes of respect for their bodies. Such a program could lead to a radical change in the fight against undetected diabetes, hypertension, eye problems and venereal disease. If the role of our schools is to prepare the young for future modern life, preventive medicine certainly has a proper place there.

3) Public information is not a medical specialty.

Therefore the job should be given to those who can do it best. I suggest that a federal agency for medical information be created with the responsibility for instructing the public on health matters. There, doctors and information specialists will work hand in hand. This agency will teach preventive medical measures to the general public, will answer public questions on health subjects and will fight unfounded health myths. Today, public medical instruction on prevention of such diseases as cancer, heart disease, hypertension and arthritis is scattered among multiple private and public associations. The creation of this specialized agency will concentrate the instructing task, will increase its efficiency and will reduce the cost.

The fight against excessive salt consumption is probably just one among many that the future holds for us. Let us be prepared with wisdom and skill. Saving life—and improving the quality of that life—is still our most human endeavor.

*Assa Weinberg, M.D.*
*New York, N.Y.*

# Peter's Story

# 2

# The First Three Weeks Are the Hardest

Living salt free and staying that way for any length of time was far from easy for me. I found it a lot harder, for example, than dieting to lose weight. That's why so many doctors seem to be skeptical about their patients being able to adhere to a low-sodium diet, except in a hospital where professional dietitians are able to control all meals. It's quite a different story in the everyday life of home and office, restaurants and parties, travel, vacations and all the other situations designed to conspire against your determination to follow a low-sodium diet.

You'll find the sodium-free variety of your favorite delicacies don't taste at all as you remember them. It seemed many of my favorite foods—cheese, cold cuts, corned beef, pastrami, Nova Scotia salmon, pickles, pretzels and peanuts—contained especially large amounts of sodium. It was the memory of those delicacies that made getting used to their low-sodium replacements quite hard. You will have to learn to acquire new tastes. Don't compare anything you eat now with what you ate before. Ease into new taste experiences gradually. Experiment with seasonings. Don't just sit back and let someone do it for you. You might even develop an interest in cooking yourself, if you don't already have one.

When you first start your diet avoid trying the salt-free versions of your favorite dishes long enough so your taste buds won't remember exactly what they tasted like. Also try to start with those that are more easily disguised by salt substitutes and sodium-free seasonings.

Here's an example: I love soup. Any kind. Any time. It gives me energy and lifts my spirit. It is also my favorite snack when I feel hungry. I was delighted when we found a whole line of canned soups all marked "for low-sodium diets" in the supermarket. I couldn't wait to get home and try one. It tasted awful. We poured in half our spice shelf. Not much of an improvement. Nothing seemed to help.

What about those dietetic bouillion cubes we had picked up? They come in beef and chicken flavor. One-half teaspoon of dehydrated soup greens, a pinch of salt substitute, two or three shakes of a seasoning called Vegit. I liked it a lot better than the canned low-sodium soups. After two or three tries we found out how to overcome some of the blandness of this homemade pick-me-up: We doubled the strength by using 2 cubes per cup. Boiling for 3 to 5 minutes brings out the full flavor of the soup greens and you have yourself a dandy dish of instant homemade vegetable soup, well within dietetic sodium levels. Naturally soup homemade from scratch will taste even better, but the principle is the same: *You have to experiment.* Venture out into the magic world of spices and try everything. Discovering how you can beat the white killer is a thrill that will turn your affliction into adventure.

Canned salmon and tuna fish salad are other favorites of mine. After not even attempting to try what their salt-free versions tasted like for several weeks we finally tackled the dietetic tuna; mixed it with salt-free mayonnaise, sliced some fresh tomato into it and with a pinch of curry, a teaspoon of lemon juice, a tablespoon of mustard oil, some frozen or dehydrated chives, plenty of dill weed, two shakes from the salt substitute shaker, it tasted fine on white toast and even better on brown untoasted bread, both salt free.

To help you keep count on your sodium intake through all this experimenting in the kitchen, consult the charts in this book.

You'll be surprised at the ever growing variety of "snack" type dietetic (in this case, low-sodium) products coming onto the market. You no longer have to be sorry for yourself at friends' parties, with everyone except you munching on pretzels and nuts. Take their salt-free version with you in a little bag and ask your hostess discreetly for a dish of your own. You'll have your hands full protecting it from nosy guests who "just want to know what it tastes like." Don't mind their derisive grimaces; it's your health you're looking after not theirs.

Speaking of parties or an invitation to a meal, discuss your diet with your hostess in advance. Find out what is being served and suggest she set aside a plate of food containing as little sodium as possible. Your expertise will come as a great relief to your hostess as she is probably anxious for you to enjoy their hospitality without endangering your health. A particularly thoughtful hostess may offer to change her entire menu because of you and then it is important that you can offer to be helpful and imaginative with alternate suggestions.

Besides the dinner recipes in this book, we have listed the best low-sodium cookbooks we could find on page 45. Your hostess may want to borrow one of them and cook a low-sodium dinner for the entire party as a novelty. Before you know it you may have started something.

After several weeks of salt-free living, your palate will have adjusted and your craving for salt will have all but subsided. Your taste buds, freed from the constant assault of salt, will stand up and salute as new hitherto unfelt taste sensations are marching by.

Various hard cheeses, pickles and mustard all now come in a low-sodium variety for the sandwich that will make you all but forget you're on a diet. The promise of a low-sodium ham by our friends at Chicago Dietetic opens up new horizons for the ubiquitous American sandwich and should give all us low-sodium dieters something to cheer about.

Thus, after a few weeks you will have adjusted to this new salt-free life, and you will have crossed over into the land of salt-free living. As you read this, it may be hard for you to imagine what that might be like, in those first difficult days of getting acquainted with the low-sodium regimen, but patience, will power and persistence mixed with a sense of adventure will make you free from salt.

There is an unexpected fringe benefit to the low-sodium diet. If you happen to be overweight and have tried in vain to lose it, this may do it. It did for me. As you cut down on your salt intake, your body will no longer retain liquid to the same extent as before. That alone will knock off a few pounds. After some weeks of sodium-free eating my taste buds started a slowdown action; I simply lost my appetite. It took no will power at all to do something I had never managed to do before—eat less. I started to look and feel younger as one inevitably does after dropping some excess weight. But there was a catch to it and I hope by passing it on to you, you will avoid it. I was concentrating so hard on trying out new low-sodium ideas, I forgot that low sodium and low calorie are not the same. Before long I started to gain weight again, and soon my weight loss, the direct result of low-sodium dieting, was wiped out—also as a direct result of low-sodium dieting. So watch out, if excess weight is one of your problems! Try to eat sensibly even when you've licked the salt problem.

# 3

# High Adventure in the Supermarket: In Search of Low-Sodium Food

As soon as I was told I would have to forego salt forever, I panicked. What would I eat? Didn't everything have salt in it? Would I have to give up all my favorites and be condemned to eating tasteless flavorless food for the rest of my life? Where were we going to find salt-free substitutes and how much more expensive would they be?

In the months to come we were amazed to see how many supermarkets and health food stores stocked salt-free products of every kind and variety, and even now the shelves of products for sodium restricted diets grow longer every day. They are usually found under "Diet Foods" and if you can't find a salt-free version of something you particularly like or want, *ask the manager.* We've tried our best to list all of the more widely marketed products in this book (pages 179–82) but your best bet is to *ask the manager.*

As we began to look more thoroughly into the salt-free scene, Dorothy's initially enthusiastic report had to be modified somewhat. Many of the products we found turned out to be second-rate. The manufacturer had done little to replace the lethal white stuff with a combination of harmless seasonings that would keep them tasty. Since taste is a very subjective matter, we can only report what, after much doctoring, appealed to us and what didn't. One thing is certain: Almost anything you can buy lends itself to a little doctoring or experimentation. We've come up with some nifty principles of seasoning, which we'll share with you in the following chapter.

I never cared much for shopping before and generally displayed a typical male chauvinist attitude toward it; from indifferent, to truculent to contemptuous. But my hypertensive affliction turned our shopping expeditions into high adventure. Dorothy returned almost daily with reports of new products much like a bird-watcher exultant at having come upon a rare species. I cruised the aisles of supermarkets like an explorer in search of buried treasure. Sometimes we could hardly wait to get into the kitchen to try out what we had found. Sometimes we were disappointed by the results. Just as often we were pleasantly surprised. A new salt substitute, a low-sodium chili that tasted surprisingly delicious. Some spice that made life worth living, even if it was salt free. Most important, with patience and persistence, we were able to find enough prepared food products to keep me on and interested in the diet, a feat most doctors regard as too difficult to try. Perhaps this explains the lack of enthusiasm some doctors show for putting their patients on this form of diet.

In those first weeks of exploration and discovery we met Sam Simon, the owner of a fancy gourmet shop called "Simon Pure," located on New York City's 57th Street. He turned out to be a good and knowledgeable friend. From him we learned some valuable general principles in our quest for low-sodium food products, and his well-stocked shelves containing a wide variety of products indicated his alertness to the growing importance of salt-free living. Mr. Sam, we discovered, was well versed in the principles of the low-sodium diet and often guided us when we found ourselves up against a new dilemma. Thus it was he who taught us that it is best to ease into the diet gradually. Some salt-free products taste delicious from the outset. Others take getting used to. Defer the latter until your palate no longer remembers what they tasted like in your salty days. Apply this "Simon says" principle to your favorite foods. Don't try to use their salt-free equivalents at once or you'll be disheartened and give up too easily. Just remember to stay within your daily sodium intake allowance! We have dealt with this principle of *adaptation* in the preceding chapter in more detail, but it is just as important to remember when you set out on your first shopping trips to stock your salt-free larder.

Not everywhere do you find gourmet shops like "Simon Pure" which stock such goodies as salt-free bouillion, cocktail crackers, catsup, cornflakes and so forth. Gourmet and health food as well as specialty stores (like cheese shops) are your best bets to find a surprising variety of low-salt or salt-free products. Also, the food and gourmet counters of the big department stores. New York City's famous Bloomingdales, for instance, sells freshly baked salt-free bread twice a week, white on Wednesdays and rye on Saturdays. And while we're on the subject of bread, don't look for the salt-free version of this staple on the bakery shelves; because it does not contain sodium it must be kept in the freezer. Among the national chains, A & P makes a good presliced white loaf under the "Ann Page" label and Freihofer's in eastern New York State supplies a fine presliced loaf of white. When you're tired of white toast, there is Wuest Soya Protein bread, presliced, a very tasty alternative, found mainly in the freezers of health food stores in the East. Our research on breads led us to conclude that this item, for which almost everyone professes to have a great fondness, is available as follows: 1) In some major food market chains, packaged and primarily white or rye. 2) In some bakeries, unsliced, freshly baked, white. 3) In many health food stores and gourmet shops, white and dark. 4) At the gourmet or delicatessen counters of department stores, often freshly baked, unsliced white and dark.

When packaged and presliced look for it in the frozen food freezers, not on the bread shelves.

Cheese lovers will be delighted to hear of an excellent Gouda imported from Holland that is available in every major cheese specialty store in almost all U.S. cities. If you can't locate it in your town, *ask the manager*. You'll be surprised what a little persistence will produce. If all else fails, write to the distributor. (We've listed as many distributors as we could find.) Find out who around your town distributes imported foods. There are also some passable salt-free cottage cheeses, which can be much improved by adding chives (fresh or dehydrated) some tomato, dill weed and a healthy dab of sour cream. We've come across a packaged Cheddar cheese in health food stores that left us less than enthusiastic. However, grilled on salt-free toast with some caraway seed and topped with a slice of tomato we found it a good between-meals-snack. Make sure it's fresh when you buy it. Its refrigerator life span is minimal (3 to 4 days). Sorry, so far no low-sodium version of our favorite, Swiss, but there is a packaged Colby cheese you might try instead.

Sometime after we had begun writing the book we discovered two excellent cheeses marketed by our friends at the Chicago Dietetic Supply Company under the "Cellu" label. Their Cheddar and Colby were steps in the right direction, but you may have to spend a little time, perhaps even write "Cellu" a letter to find out where you can get them. You'll find the address on page 179.

Many products essential to salt-free living will not be located on the diet food sections, nor do you have to look for them in health, gourmet or specialty shops. Butter and margarine, for example, are available almost everywhere in unsalted as well as salted versions. So are matzos, the unleavened bread associated with the Jewish festival of Passover, but you don't have to be Jewish to consume it in all shapes and sizes and on all occasions. It makes an excellent dietary substitute for bread or salted crackers and is available in an unsalted version year-round. So are unsalted, roasted peanuts, and, by the time you read this, half a dozen other products.

Which brings us to an essential commandment of those having to live the salt-free life: *Read all labels carefully.* Some manufacturers are not too precise about listing the sodium content of their products, others disguise it or make it tough for the uninitiated to understand. The sodium content of any prepared food should be listed on the package in milligrams, which is abbreviated like this: "mgs." When you see something listed like this "0.5 gms." that actually means 500 mgs. While this looks like very little, it's the works on a daily diet of 500 mgs., which is the average daily sodium intake a doctor has in mind when he puts you on a low-sodium diet.

Just as important for you is that labels should show the per unit sodium content of what's inside the package. Thus, "per tspn." or "per oz." or "per cup" is essential for you to know if you are to keep track of how much sodium you are taking in per day.

At present, we found labeling for sodium content to be haphazard to say the least and a fertile field for consumer advocates to look into. And while we're on the subject of consumerism, your pursuit of salt-free happiness will lead you to the discovery that salt-free and low-sodium products are more expensive than their regular counterparts. Those, who on their doctor's orders have to live a salt-free life, may as well face the fact that while their blood pressure may come down, their food bills will go up.

In canned foods one name reigns supreme: Chicago Dietetic's "Featherweight" is by far the most diversified and widely distributed manufacturer of products for low-sodium diets. Many of their products are also marketed under the "Cellu" label. They were the pioneers in this business and continue to bring out new items each year. We found them knowledgeable and dedicated to overcoming the central problem of the low-sodium diet: blandness. Another important name to remember is that of California's Tillie Lewis who specializes in canned vegetables, soups and juices. So does Balanced Foods of New Jersey. More and more manufacturers appear on the supermarket shelves with salt-free versions of their products: S&W under the "Nutradiet" label; Campbell's soups have come out with low-sodium versions of their product but in my opinion you'll have to give your spice shelf quite a workout before their soups taste as if they weren't part of the menu in a maximum security institution.

On almost every dietetic food shelf you'll find an array of salt substitutes by various commercial manufacturers. Morton's, in containers almost indistinguishable from their regular shakers (we think this is both foolish and misleading since the person having to use the substitute could easily confuse it with its regular salt dispensers).

While all of them are more or less the same, some tasted "saltier" than others. I particularly liked Neocurtesal, obtainable only in drugstores. Ask your druggist what else he sells as a salt substitute for sodium restricted diets. You may discover something more to your liking. Be sure to test any salt substitute before you use it in cooking, as all of them contain a large amount of potassium which tends to taste bitter when heated. To avoid this it is best added at the table.

Whenever Dorothy and I visit a new place, we head for the nearest supermarket. A quick survey of the diet food shelves tells us how hip its manager is about low-sodium food. A brief interview with him tells us more and tells him there are people who will buy salt-free products, if he decides to stock them. A visit to two or three bakeries, the local health food, cheese and gourmet stores and a delicatessen and we're all set. If you follow this simple procedure you, too, can turn shopping for salt-free food from a chore into an adventure.

# 4

# Cooking Without Salt— A Challenge to Your Imagination and Resourcefulness

Cooking salt free depends on your approach to cooking generally: whether you regard it as a chore or a way to express yourself. To Dorothy and myself it is a challenge. It consists mainly of finding the right kind of substitutes for salt; of enhancing prepared foods and creating taste sensations that make me forget I am on a diet. Since both of us love to putter around in the kitchen and neither of us is intimidated by cookbooks, measuring cups or scales, we took up the challenge of low-sodium cooking with the enthusiastic abandon of a four-year-old discovering finger painting.

Dorothy maintains that my sharing her interest in mastering the low-sodium cuisine has a lot to do with my ability to stay on this diet. Indeed here, I think, she has hit upon an important principle of all dieting: persons on any kind of diet should not just be served dietetic food or told what they can or cannot eat. Instead they should become *involved* in preparing, testing, experimenting and solving the special problems connected with the diet. Chances are their involvement and their conversion from passive "victim" to active participant will help them maintain considerably more interest in adhering to a regime that requires will power and self-discipline.

Cooking, we believe, is a highly creative form of

self-expression that requires both skill and natural inclination. It can be learned up to a point, but from then on it is sheer inspiration. If cooking is not your thing, the need to prepare sodium restricted dishes is certainly not going to turn you into a gourmet chef. Since there are already a good many cookbooks for sodium-restricted diets we have simply listed them at the end of this chapter in what we felt was the order of importance, realizing that here, too, personal preference can make for wide differences of opinion. Some people like chatty cookbooks, others prefer the nitty-gritty type and others still go for the inventive or innovative ones. Our list includes whatever we could find because at the time we needed them, low-sodium cookbooks were still relatively hard to find. We feel confident that as low-sodium diets are more widely prescribed, more and better low-sodium cookbooks will come onto the market.

Sometimes neither of our careers permit us the luxury of spending hours in the kitchen to prepare different meals for all members of our lively household (two teenage daughters, a poodle, a proliferating family of tropical fish, a "sleep-over" child perhaps, and—when we spend weekends at our house in the country—a guest or two or more). Frequently we simply don't have the time to prepare every meal from the ground up, so we have tried to share with you our experience of preparing some basic dishes and doctoring prepared foods.

First, take a good look at your spice shelf and if you don't have one get a good one quickly. A good spice shelf should contain all the standard and some exotic spices in clearly marked glass containers that close hermetically. They should be displayed so that their names are easily visible, preferably near where you do your cooking and where you can reach them effortlessly. If you need some help, there is the American Spice Trade Association in the Empire State Building, New York City, N.Y. 10001, which will be glad to send you all kinds of helpful reading material on seasoning your low-sodium food. So will one of the leading spice traders, "McCormick," whose products are found extensively in supermarkets throughout the U.S. and Canada, as are "Ehler's" whose dehydrated soup greens and many other seasonings we found extremely good and helpful. A Home Economics director named "Mary Collins" presides over McCormick's test kitchens and was most informative and knowledgeable when we wrote to her. We are not suggesting for a moment that all information obtained from commercial sources should be accepted on face value, but we have tested enough samples to feel reasonably confident that most of the information on sodium content supplied by reputable manufacturers is fairly accurate. (See pages 179–82 for addresses.)

One suggestion appealed to us particularly, because it allowed our creativity and imagination to run rampant: Forever interested in promoting the sale of spices, the Spice Traders Association gave us the idea of blending those spices that especially beguile our taste buds and of keeping on hand a shakerful of our own blend to use at home or carry with us when we eat out.

Almost all low-sodium prepared food products can do with healthy helpings of seasoning to give them taste appeal. However, since taste varies greatly from person to person, it is here that you have the greatest opportunity to experiment and give free reign to your own imagination and sense of adventure.

We have found several herbs and spices particularly effective in replacing salt: dill weed, curry, pepper, paprika, garlic powder (not garlic salt!) and onion powder (not onion salt!) are my favorites and dehydrated chives and parsley run a close second. Some others are not so easy to find and you may have to write to their manufacturers to find out which of the stores in your neighborhood carries them. One is an all-purpose seasoning called "Vegit" (by Modern Products Inc. of Milwaukee, Wisconsin 53209). Its sodium content is relatively high, but since the amounts of it you will add to your food are very small, it will not seriously effect your D.S.I. (daily sodium intake). The other, a bacon seasoning that's great with eggs, salads and some meats, is called "Hickory Smoked Yeast" by Sovex of White Plains, N.Y., which I discovered on my periodic explorations to that best of dietetic gourmet shops, "Simon Pure" of New York City. And there is always Chicago Dietetic, who come out with a new low-sodium product of superior quality practically every month, mostly under the "Featherweight" label.

Sherry and cooking wines add considerable zest to many dishes that would otherwise taste bland without salt, and can be of considerable help in livening up a dinner party, something salt could never do.

Vegetables vary greatly in sodium content. The frozen packed ones say "Lightly Salted" or "Salt Added," but if you are on a minimum D.S.I. diet, you ought to be careful and check our charts, for the fresh as well as frozen or canned variety.

Salad dressings are available in sodium-free and low-calorie versions by now (here, too, "Featherweight" shines!). Personally I like to make my own dressing. To give it some oomph I prefer to use flavored oils and vinegars, like mustard oil, garlic oil, sesame oil, tarragon and red wine vinegars. I add a healthy dash of salad herbs. (We use "Ehlers" but I am sure there are all kinds. Just read the label on the container carefully, to make sure it contains no salt.)

Desserts, sodas, cookies and ice cream all contain amounts of sodium and our charts will help you stay within your daily sodium intake.

Bread and butter or margarine are no longer hard to get rarities. In our chapter on shopping and in the sample menus, we have dealt with these items and all other food products we could possibly think of. If we have missed one and you discover it, write to us, care of our publisher, Bantam Books, 666 Fifth Avenue, New York City, N.Y. 10019 so it can be included in the next edition.

Cooking for the low-sodium (sodium restricted) diet can be summed up like this:

1. Use low-sodium raw materials (fresh vegetables, fruits, meats and fish).
2. Buy only low-sodium prepared foods.
3. Learn all you can about spices and seasonings.
4. Keep your eyes open for new products when you go shopping.
5. Read all labels very carefully.
6. Plan your daily menus with the help of our charts at the end of this book.

Gourmet cooks should start a collection of low-sodium cookbooks. We've listed below those we have found.

## Low sodium cookbooks

*Salt Free Cooking with Herbs and Spices* by June Roth. Chicago: Henry Regnery, 1975.

*Cooking Without A Grain of Salt* by Elma W. Bagg. New York: Bantam Books, 1972.

*Living Salt Free and Easy* by Anna Houston Thorburn with Phyllis Turner. Los Angeles: Douglas-West Publishers, 1975.

*The Salt-Free Diet Cookbook* by Emil G. Conason, M.D. and Ella Metz. New York: Grosset & Dunlap, 1969.

There'll be others and the growing popularity of salt-free eating will lead to new ones as time goes on.

In the beginning you may prefer simple preparations and dishes that are easy and quick to prepare. Our suggestions for that period until you yourself are ready to meet the low-sodium challenge follow.

In the pages that follow we have described how certain categories of food should be cooked the salt-free way. They are simple recipes designed to illustrate the principles of salt-free cooking. We hope they will serve to inspire you when you try to create your own recipes.

# 5

# Recipes

## Cereals

For extra flavor in preparing salt-free hot cereals, add salt-free margarine or butter while cooking and flavor with brown sugar, cinnamon or honey. (There is a low-calorie brown sugar for those who must restrict their sugar intake). Fresh fruits of all kinds can be served with both hot and cold cereals to liven up their flavor.

## Desserts

Desserts are indeed easy as so many fruits are low in sodium and can be used in so many different ways. Fruits can be served fresh, stewed, baked or sauced, and there are the canned and frozen varieties also. Good puddings and gelatins that are low-sodium dietary are also available. Even applesauce can be made more interesting by adding currants and cinnamon in the cooking, and by cooking the apples in their skin and straining them along with the cooked currants. To dress up desserts (they should be festive) we suggest the following ideas:

## GRAND MARNIER FRUIT SUPREME

1 medium grapefruit, sectioned
2 medium oranges, sectioned
2 cups melon balls (unsweetened frozen or fresh cantaloupe and honeydew)
½ cup sliced strawberries or raspberries (unsweetened frozen or fresh)
½ cup blueberries (unsweetened frozen or fresh)
1 cup pineapple chunks with juice (canned unsweetened)
2 jiggers (3 ounces) Grand Marnier

Combine the fruits in a large bowl with their natural juices. Add the Grand Marnier and mix very gently. Cover and refrigerate overnight.

*7 mg per serving* *Serves 8–10*

## CRÈME DE MENTHE PEARS

4 pears, peeled, halved and cored
1 cup water
2 tablespoons sugar or an equivalent amount of sugar substitute
2 tablespoons crème de menthe

Simmer pears in water and sugar in a covered pot until soft. Allow to cool. When cold add crème de menthe to the cooking liquid. Pour over the pears and refrigerate at least 3 hours before serving.

*5 mg per serving* *Serves 4*

# Eggs

Eggs are generally easy to prepare salt free. Soft boiled, poached, and hard boiled never have salt added in their preparation and fried or scrambled can be cooked in salt-free butter or margarine. Salt substitute can be added as desired after cooking. Even omelets and French toast can be prepared salt free. Chives, dehydrated minced onion, chervil, paprika, oregano, savory, tarragon, and a bacon flavored Hickory Smoked Yeast (by Sovex) can be used to help you prepare many different kinds of omelets. Jelly, jam and fruit omelets are also quite delicious. Here are a few examples to help you get started in creating your own recipes.

### BACON FLAVORED WESTERN OMELET

½ teaspoon Hickory Flavored Yeast (Sovex)
1 egg
1 teaspoon chopped onion or ¼ teaspoon dehydrated onion
1 tablespoon diced tomato
1 teaspoon diced green pepper
1 teaspoon salt-free butter, margarine or greaseless frying product
Pepper

Add Hickory Flavored Yeast to egg and beat. Stir in onions, tomato and green pepper. Pour mixture into a greased pan. Season lightly with pepper. Cover with lid and cook on medium flame until done.

*60 mg per serving* *Serves 1*

### CHEESE 'N CHIVE OMELET

1 egg
1 teaspoon chopped chives (dehydrated or fresh)
1 teaspoon salt-free butter, margarine or greaseless frying product
¼ teaspoon grated Parmesan cheese
Pepper

Beat egg. Add chives and pour into greased pan. Sprinkle lightly with grated cheese and pepper. Cover with lid and cook on medium flame until done.

*65 mg per serving* *Serves 1*

### LOW-SODIUM FRENCH TOAST

1 egg
⅛ teaspoon vanilla
⅓ cup low-sodium milk (diluted)
1 teaspoon sugar or an equivalent amount of sugar substitute
¼ teaspoon nutmeg
2 slices low-sodium bread
1 tablespoon salt-free butter or margarine
½ teaspoon cinnamon

Beat egg. Add vanilla, milk, sugar, and nutmeg. Soak bread in the mixture. On a griddle, brown bread in the butter, turning once. Sprinkle with cinnamon. Serve with honey or low-sodium jam.

*66 mg per serving* *Serves 1*

## Fish

As broiled fish must be cooked just before eating, it is a good dish to order when eating out. It is easy to request that it be prepared without salt. Fresh lemon juice will enhance its taste. When cooking at home you can add spices, herbs, wine and use the various low-sodium cream sauces we have suggested. Garlic, cumin, mace, dill, curry, parsley and turmeric are some of the herbs and spices that can be used. Onions, tomatoes and green peppers are also helpful to enhance the natural flavor of the fish. Since broiling fish is relatively quick and easy, it is a good place for the "noncook" dieter to become involved in experimenting with different seasonings. Their involvement in the preparation is an important factor in sustaining the will to diet. Here are a few of the results of our experiments.

### HALIBUT BAKED WITH DILL SAUCE

1 teaspoon lemon juice
2 teaspoons melted salt-free butter or margarine
2 halibut steaks
1 cup Creamed Dill Sauce (see p. 62)
Pepper
Parsley
Lemon slices

Add lemon juice to the melted butter. Brush both sides of the halibut with the butter and allow it to soak in for a few minutes. Place halibut in a baking dish and pour over Creamed Dill Sauce. Bake at 350°F for about 20 minutes, or until fish flakes easily when tested with a fork. Garnish with parsley, pepper and a slice of lemon.

*91 mg per serving* *Serves 2*

## BAKED RED SNAPPER

6 tablespoons salt-free butter or margarine
½ cup chopped onion
2 cups diced tomatoes
¼ cup chopped green pepper
1 tablespoon low-sodium chili sauce
1 teaspoon chili powder
1 teaspoon lemon juice
2 bay leaves
½ teaspoon oregano
⅛ teaspoon white pepper
1 (4-pound) red snapper

Melt butter. Add onion, tomatoes, green pepper, chili sauce, chili powder, lemon juice, bay leaves, oregano and pepper. Stir until ingredients are blended and simmer until tender. Place fish in a baking pan. Pour sauce over and bake at 350°F for about 45 minutes, basting frequently with the sauce.

*215 mg per serving* *Serves 6*

## CURRIED SHRIMP

1 pound shrimp, peeled and deveined
2 tablespoons cooking oil
1 cup Creamed Curry Sauce (see p.62)

In heavy skillet cook shrimps quickly in hot oil, stirring frequently. Heat Creamed Curry Sauce in saucepan. When shrimps are cooked, drain excess oil and add shrimps to sauce. Simmer for 2 or 3 minutes and serve.

*232 mg per serving* *Serves 4*

## SHRIMP SCAMPI

1 pound shrimp, peeled and deveined
2 tablespoons cooking oil
1 teaspoon garlic powder

Season shrimps with garlic. In heavy skillet cook quickly in hot oil, stirring frequently. Can be served with additional salt-free garlic butter sauce.

*215 mg per serving* *Serves 4*

## Hors d'oeuvres and snacks

There are enough salt-free crackers on the market for everyone to find one that they enjoy. Tuna, salmon and egg salad spreads (for our salt-free version, see p. 60) as well as low-sodium cheeses can be used on the crackers. Of course, there is a large selection of salt-free nuts, potato chips, potato sticks, sesame sticks and pretzels. Raw vegetable sticks with our salt-free dip may inspire you to create some dips of your own.

### GRILLED CHEESE

1 ounce low-sodium cheese, sliced
1 slice low-sodium white bread
1 slice tomato
¼ teaspoon caraway seeds

Place cheese on bread and top with tomato. Sprinkle with caraway seeds. Place under broiler until bread toasts and cheese bubbles.

*13 mg per serving* *Serves 1*

### EGGS À LA RUSSE

2 tablespoons low-sodium mayonnaise
2 tablespoons low-sodium chili sauce
¼ teaspoon paprika
½ teaspoon oregano
Dash of pepper
2 hard-boiled eggs
4 large lettuce leaves

Combine mayonnaise, chili sauce, paprika, oregano and pepper and blend until smooth. Slice each egg in half. Arrange on lettuce leaves. Divide mayonnaise mixture evenly between egg halves and chill.

*35 mg per serving* *Serves 4*

### DEVILED EGGS

4 hard-boiled eggs
4 teaspoons low-sodium mayonnaise
4 teaspoons low-sodium mustard
¼ teaspoon paprika

Cut eggs in half, remove yolks and mash. Add mayonnaise and mustard and blend until smooth. Put egg mixture back into the egg whites. Garnish with paprika and serve.

*32 mg per ½ egg* *Serves 4–8*

**DIP FOR RAW VEGETABLES**

4 tablespoons sour cream
½ cup low-sodium cottage cheese
1 tablespoon dehydrated onion
¼ teaspoon curry powder
1 teaspoon low-sodium mustard
1 teaspoon lemon juice
½ teaspoon paprika
Pepper

Blend the above ingredients until mixture is fairly smooth.

*(76 mg for entire dip)*

**RAW VEGETABLES**

8 (4-inch) carrot sticks
10 radishes
1 cup cauliflower flowerets
1 green pepper, sliced into strips
2 broccoli stalks

*(107 mg for all vegetables)*
*31 mg per serving* *Serves 6*

## Meats

Meats are generally easy to deal with. Garlic, paprika and pepper can be used to flavor for broiling and roasting. Steaks broiled with garlic and salt-free margarine or butter, lamb roasted with garlic cloves, lamb chops broiled with paprika and roast beef prepared with pepper and paprika can satisfy the fussiest eater. As in any kind of cooking, the quality of the meat is the most important element. There are a myriad of recipes for all kinds of salt-free ways to prepare meat dishes. The following are some of the results of our salt-free cooking experiences.

## POT ROAST

4 pounds chuck, round or rump of beef
1 garlic clove, halved
2 tablespoons fat
3 medium-sized onions, coarsely chopped
2 tomatoes, diced
¼ cup low-sodium tomato juice
3 marrow bones
2 bay leaves
Pepper
½ teaspoon paprika
¼ teaspoon thyme

Rub the meat with garlic clove. In a Dutch oven brown the meat on all sides in the fat. Remove the meat and brown the onions. Then add tomatoes (with liquid), tomato juice, marrow bones and bay leaves. Season the meat with pepper and paprika and return to the pot. Sprinkle in thyme. Cover pot tightly and simmer gently for 3 to 4 hours, or until done. Make sure that there is always ½ inch of liquid in the pot. If roast becomes dry, add low-sodium tomato juice.

There are variations of the above recipe. For example: (1) the meat can be marinated overnight in wine, bay leaves and spices, and this stock used in the above recipe instead of the tomatoes and tomato juice. (2) Vegetables such as carrots, potatoes and fresh string beans can be added to the pot in the last hour of cooking. (Add the string beans last if you like them slightly underdone.)

*67 mg per serving (without vegetables)* *Serves 6–8*

## BAKED PORK CHOPS WITH CARROTS AND PINEAPPLE

8 carrots, cut into 4-inch sticks
8 thinly sliced pork chops
¼ teaspoon garlic powder
1 (6-ounce) can unsweetened frozen orange juice concentrate
1 (20-ounce) can unsweetened pineapple chunks
2 tablespoons brown sugar or an equivalent amount of sugar substitute
½ teaspoon nutmeg

Place carrots in a Dutch oven or covered casserole. Sprinkle pork chops lightly with garlic powder and place on top of the carrots. Mix the undiluted orange juice with the juice from the pineapple chunks. Add brown sugar and nutmeg to the mixture. Pour mixture over pork chops and carrots. Cover and bake at 450°F. After 1 hour turn pork chops over. When almost done add the pineapple chunks.

*123 mg per serving* *Serves 4*

## BEEF STEW BURGUNDY

2 pounds cubed beef for stew (lean)
2 small onions, diced
1 tablespoon oil
6 carrots, peeled and cut into 4-inch sticks
6 small potatoes, peeled
4 small whole onions
½ teaspoon thyme
½ teaspoon oregano
½ teaspoon garlic powder
Pepper
½ teaspoon paprika
1 cup Burgundy cooking wine
1 pound green beans, whole, trimmed

In a skillet brown meat and diced onions lightly in oil. Transfer to a large Dutch oven and add carrots, potatoes and whole onions. Add thyme, oregano, garlic powder, pepper and paprika to wine, mix and pour half of it over meat and vegetables. Cover tightly and bake at 400°F until meat is tender, 2 to 3 hours. About 30 minutes before serving add the green beans and pour the rest of the wine mixture over them.

*100 mg per serving* *Serves 6*

## Pastas and Rice

If you refer to the charts in the back of the book, rice and pasta are salt-free unless salt is added in the cooking. Spaghetti, cooked in water with lemon juice, served with garlic and oil is delicious and salt free as well. There is a prepared low-sodium tomato sauce that can be perked up with spices and herbs as well as a low-sodium canned Spanish rice. Here's a rice dish that is a little bit different and is appropriately served with a curry dish.

## RICE WITH RAISINS AND ALMONDS

1 cup uncooked rice
1 cup orange juice
1¼ cups water
¼ cup golden raisins
1 tablespoon brown sugar or an equivalent amount of sugar substitute
¼ teaspoon ginger
1 tablespoon salt-free margarine or butter
½ cup chopped almonds
½ teaspoon cinnamon

Combine rice, orange juice, water, raisins, sugar, ginger and margarine in a saucepan and bring to a full boil. Reduce heat and simmer, covered, for about 15 minutes, or until soft. Remove from the heat and allow to stand for 8 minutes. Sprinkle with almonds and cinnamon and serve hot.

*5 mg per serving* *Serves 4*

## TUNA-NOODLE CASSEROLE

This tuna casserole is another idea for disguising the blandness of noodles cooked without salt.

9 tablespoons powdered low-sodium milk (undiluted)
6 tablespoons salt-free mayonnaise
2 tablespoons dehydrated chopped onion
Pepper
1 tablespoon lemon juice
3 tablespoons salt-free margarine
1 cup water
1 (8-ounce) package noodles
½ teaspoon garlic powder
1 cup fresh peas, cooked
1 (7-ounce) can low-sodium tuna, flaked
1 teaspoon grated Parmesan cheese

Mix powdered milk, mayonnaise, onion, pepper, margarine, lemon juice and water in a blender. Cook noodles according to package directions, undercooking slightly and using garlic in the water instead of salt. Drain. Put cooked noodles, cooked peas and tuna in a casserole and pour blended mixture over it. Sprinkle top lightly with Parmesan cheese and bake at 450°F for 30 minutes or until lightly brown.

*26 mg per serving* *Serves 6–8*

NOTE: The Parmesan cheese used in the recipe is high in sodium, but because it is used in such a small quantity it adds very little to the total sodium content of the recipe. However, it is important not to vary the amount of cheese used.

## Poultry

Chicken, turkey, duck and other poultry are exceedingly tasty in their salt-free versions. Chicken and turkey roasted with garlic, pepper and paprika are just fine, and chicken broiled with salt-free butter or margarine, garlic, pepper and paprika will satisfy even someone not on a low-sodium regime. Potted chicken has been described in the section on soup (see page 65). Poultry cooked with fruits are particularly tasty and fun to invent. My teenage daughter Carrie devised the following recipe.

### CHICKEN À L'ORANGE

- ½ teaspoon poultry seasoning
- 1 (4-pound) roasting chicken
- 1 (3-ounce) can frozen unsweetened orange juice concentrate
- 2 tablespoons whole cranberry sauce or diet cranberry sauce
- ¼ teaspoon ginger
- 2 tablespoons brown sugar or an equivalent amount of sugar substitute

Sprinkle poultry seasoning on all sides of the chicken. Mix orange juice concentrate, cranberry sauce, ginger and sugar. Blend well. Coat chicken with mixture.

Bake at 325°F for about 1½ to 2 hours, or until tender. Keep basting with fruit mixture.

This recipe can be used with other fowl such as duck, capon, etc., varying the cooking time and the temperature of the oven.

*96 mg per serving* *Serves 4*

## Salads

There are many vegetables and fruits to choose from in making salads, and there are diverse low-sodium prepared dressings (see p. 63). We make our own low-sodium Russian dressing (see p. 63). The different kinds of oils, vinegars, spices, herbs and lemon juice lend themselves to preparing dressings to suit your own particular taste.

We have included a few examples of different kinds of salad; main dish salads, side dish salads and salad spreads. Don't forget that pepper and salt substitute can be used when serving and a slice of lemon or a sprig of parsley served as a garnish enhances any salad.

### CHEF SALAD

1 clove garlic
1 small head lettuce
2 hard-boiled eggs, sliced
½ cucumber, peeled and sliced
4 radishes, sliced
½ green pepper, sliced
3 ounces cold turkey strips
2 ounces cold roast beef strips
2 tomatoes, quartered
2 ounces low-sodium cheese strips
Russian dressing (see p. 63)
Freshly ground pepper

Rub salad bowl with garlic. Arrange lettuce, eggs, cucumber, radishes, green pepper, turkey, roast beef, tomatoes and cheese. Serve with dressing and sprinkle with freshly ground pepper.

*69 mg per salad serving* *Serves 4*
*5 mg per tablespoon dressing*

## CHICKEN DELIGHT

- 3 tablespoons low-sodium mayonnaise
- 1 teaspoon salad herbs
- ¼ teaspoon garlic powder
- ½ celery stalk, finely chopped
- ½ teaspoon nutmeg
- 2 tablespoons chopped golden raisins
- 2 teaspoons lemon juice
- Pepper
- 1 cup diced chicken
- ½ cup peeled, diced apples
- 2 walnuts, chopped
- Sliced fresh pineapple
- Boston lettuce
- Cinnamon

Mix mayonnaise, herbs, garlic, celery, nutmeg, raisins, lemon juice and pepper. Add chicken and blend well. Add apples and nuts and toss lightly. Arrange chicken salad and pineapple on lettuce and sprinkle with cinnamon.

*71 mg per serving* *Serves 3*

## MANDARIN ORANGE SALAD

- Mandarine oranges
- Boston lettuce
- Shredded onions or chopped scallions
- Oil
- Vinegar
- Lemon juice
- Rosemary
- Parsley

Arrange mandarin oranges on Boston lettuce. Sprinkle with onions or scallions. Mix 3 parts oil to 1 part vinegar. Add 1 teaspoon lemon juice and ¼ teaspoon rosemary for each half cup of dressing. Garnish with a sprig of parsley.

*Less than 5 mg per serving*

## CUCUMBER SALAD

2 large cucumbers
¼ cup tarragon vinegar
¼ teaspoon garlic powder
½ teaspoon dehydrated dill weed or fresh chopped dill
½ teaspoon lemon juice
Pepper
1 tablespoon sour cream

Peel cucumbers and slice very thin. Mix vinegar, garlic, dill, lemon juice and a dash of pepper. Pour mixture over cucumbers and cover. Refrigerate for 24 hours. Drain off some of the liquid and add the sour cream before serving.

*5 mg per serving* *Serves 6*

## COLESLAW

1 teaspoon dry mustard
2 teaspoons sugar or an equivalent amount of sugar substitute
2 tablespoons flour
¼ teaspoon paprika
½ cup water
1 whole egg
¼ cup vinegar
2 tablespoons salt-free butter or margarine
2 tablespoons sour cream
1 small head cabbage, shredded

Dissolve the mustard, sugar, flour and paprika in water. Beat egg and vinegar in the top of a double boiler. Add the dissolved ingredients. Cook, stirring, over boiling water until thick and smooth. Add butter. Remove from heat and chill. Mix in the sour cream. Pour on the cabbage and toss. Salt-substitute should be added when serving.

*65 mg per cup* *Serves 4*

## PICKLED BEET SALAD

- 1/4 cup distilled vinegar
- 1/4 cup beet juice (from low-sodium beets)
- 2 teaspoons sugar or an equivalent amount of sugar substitute
- 1 (8-ounce) can low-sodium beets
- 1/2 small onion, finely sliced
- 1/2 teaspoon pickling spices

Pour vinegar, beet juice and sugar over beets, onions and pickling spices. Cover and refrigerate for at least 24 hours.

*20 mg per serving* *Serves 6*

## EGG SALAD SPREAD

Cold low-sodium Creamed Onion Sauce, Creamed Curry Sauce and Creamed Dill Sauce (see p. 62) can be used with hard-boiled eggs to make a variety of egg salad spreads. Mash eggs and sauce together in the proportion of 1 tablespoon sauce for each hard-boiled egg. When serving, season to taste with salt substitute.

*Approximately 65 mg per egg*

## EGG SALAD PLATE

Arrange Egg Salad Spread on leaves of Boston lettuce with a quartered tomato and 1/2 shredded carrot. Garnish with a sprig of parsley.

## SALMON SALAD SPREAD

- 1 (3 1/2-ounce) can low-sodium salmon, drained
- 2 tablespoons low-sodium Creamed Dill Sauce (see p. 62)
- Paprika
- Salt substitute

Flake salmon. Add sauce and mix well until smooth. Garnish with paprika and season to taste with salt substitute.

*78 mg per serving*

## SALMON SALAD PLATE

Arrange Salmon Salad Spread on lettuce with thinly sliced cucumber, tomato and onion.

## TUNA SALAD SPREAD

1 (3½-ounce) can low-sodium tuna fish, drained
2 tablespoons salt-free mayonnaise
1 teaspoon vinegar
2 tablespoons lemon juice
2 teaspoons dehydrated onion
¼ teaspoon curry powder
Pepper
Salt substitute

Flake tuna fish for easy mixing. Add mayonnaise, vinegar, lemon juice, onion, curry powder and a dash of pepper. Mix until smooth. Garnish with paprika. Season to taste with salt substitute.

*53 mg per serving* *Serves 1*

## TUNA SALAD PLATE

Scoop out the center of a tomato. Fill the inside of the tomato with Tuna Salad Spread. Place stuffed tomato on a bed of lettuce surrounding it with slices of green pepper and radishes.

## Sauces and Dressings

Sauces and dressings should be prepared in advance and refrigerated. Heated they are good to enhance the taste of a vegetable or fish. Using these sauces in different ways you can create your own recipes. Cold, they can be mixed with salmon or eggs to make various spreads. They also can be used as a base for the Tuna-Noodle Casserole (see p. 55) or Curried Shrimp (see p. 50).

## CREAMED CURRY SAUCE

9 tablespoons low-sodium milk powder
6 tablespoons low-sodium mayonnaise
3 tablespoons salt-free margarine
2 to 3 teaspoons curry powder
1 tablespoon lemon juice
1 cup water
Pepper

Put milk powder, mayonnaise, margarine, curry powder, lemon juice, water and pepper in a blender and blend until smooth. Simmer mixture over a low heat until smooth and thick. Can be used hot or can be refrigerated for later use.

*57 mg per cup* *Yields 1½ cups*

## CREAMED DILL SAUCE

9 tablespoons low-sodium milk powder
6 tablespoons low-sodium mayonnaise
3 tablespoons salt-free margarine
4 teaspoons chopped dill weed
1 tablespoon lemon juice
1 cup water
Pepper

Put milk powder, mayonnaise, margarine, dill, lemon juice, water and pepper in a blender and blend until smooth. Simmer mixture over a low heat until smooth and thick. Can be used hot or refrigerated for later use.

*58 mg per cup* *Yields 1½ cups*

## CREAMED ONION SAUCE

9 tablespoons low-sodium milk powder
6 tablespoons low-sodium mayonnaise
3 tablespoons salt-free margarine
1 tablespoon dehydrated chopped onion
1 tablespoon lemon juice
1 cup water
Pepper

Put milk powder, mayonnaise, margarine, onion, lemon juice, water and pepper in a blender and blend until smooth. Simmer mixture over a low flame until smooth and thick. Can be used hot or can be refrigerated for later use.

*63 mg per cup* *Yields 1½ cups*

**RUSSIAN DRESSING**

Low-sodium mayonnaise
Low-sodium chili sauce
Garlic powder
Pepper
McCormick's Italian Seasoning herbs

Mix equal parts of mayonnaise and chili sauce. For each cup of dressing add ¼ teaspoon garlic powder, a pinch of pepper and ½ teaspoon of Italian seasoning herbs. Blend thoroughly.

*5 mg per tablespoon*

**SEAFOOD COCKTAIL SAUCE**

Low-sodium mayonnaise
Low-sodium chili sauce
Chili powder
Tabasco sauce
Pepper

Mix equal parts of mayonnaise and chili sauce. Add chili powder, Tabasco and freshly ground pepper to taste. Blend until smooth.

*5 mg per tablespoon*

## Soups

Soup used to be a NO on salt-free diets. You no longer have to deprive yourself of this important "pick-me-up" food. A great variety of canned soups have been created in their salt-free versions. However, they do need the addition of spices and herbs. There are also many soups one can make from scratch that you will find in the various cookbooks on the market.

For "quick soups" we suggest the following ways of using low-sodium prepared soups. We've also included our favorite old-fashioned chicken soup.

## CREAMED TOMATO SOUP

1 can low-sodium condensed tomato soup
½ can Creamed Onion Sauce (see p. 62)
½ can water
2 tablespoons cooking sherry
½ teaspoon dehydrated chives
Salt substitute

Combine soup, sauce and water. Bring to a boil, stirring until smooth. Reduce heat. Add sherry and chives. Simmer 2 to 3 minutes. When serving, season to taste with salt substitute.
*39 mg per serving* *Serves 2*

## VEGETABLE SOUP

1 can low-sodium condensed vegetable soup
1 can water
¼ teaspoon Vegit
2 tablespoons cooking sherry
1 teaspoon lemon juice
Salt substitute

Bring soup, water and Vegit to a boil, slowly stirring until thoroughly mixed. Add sherry and lemon juice and simmer for 2 to 3 minutes. When serving, season to taste with salt substitute.
*19 mg per serving* *Serves 2*

## PETER'S QUICK "PICK-ME-UP" SOUP

2 low-sodium bouillon cubes
1 cup water
½ teaspoon dehydrated soup greens
¼ teaspoon Vegit
Salt substitute

Dissolve bouillon cubes in water adding soup greens and Vegit. Bring to a boil and then simmer for 3 to 5 minutes. Season to taste with salt substitute and serve hot.

*36 mg per serving* *Serves 1*

## DOROTHY'S CHICKEN SOUP

1 (4–5 pound) chicken, quartered and cleaned
4 carrots, peeled and cut into 4-inch lengths
4 celery stalks, cut into 4-inch lengths plus the leaves
4 parsnips, scraped and cut into 4-inch lengths
2 turnips, quartered
4 small onions
2 scallions, minced
1 bunch parsley sprigs, dill and other greens
Pepper
Salt substitute
2 quarts water
Remove as much fat as possible and reserve the giblets

Combine chicken, giblets, carrots, celery, parsnips, turnips, onions, scallions, greens, pepper and water in a large pot. Simmer for about 3 hours, or until chicken is tender. Allow it to cool with all of the ingredients in it and then strain out the soup. Place soup in a separate container and chill. The excess fat will rise to the top and can be easily removed. When serving, season to taste with salt substitute.

*150 mg per serving, including soup, chicken and all vegetables* *Serves 6*

## Vegetables

Vegetables served without salt actually improves everyone's eating habits. First of all, adding salt while cooking vegetables tends to remove some of their vitamin content. Also, cooking without salt will inspire you to bring out the taste of vegetables instead of hiding it. Steaming vegetables in water with a small amount of garlic powder brings out the natural flavor of a vegetable rather than giving it a garlic taste. Here are just a few of the possible ways to deal with vegetables. You'll be able to create dozens more with spices and herbs such as chives, dill weed, garlic, marjoram, oregano, pepper, savory, tarragon, thyme and turmeric. Some vegetables, such as peas or carrots, are greatly enhanced by sugar, nutmeg or cinnamon.

### BROCCOLI WITH SESAME

- 8 ounces broccoli, cut into 2-inch pieces
- 2 tablespoons cooking oil
- 1 tablespoon sesame oil
- ½ teaspoon sesame seeds

Stir-fry broccoli in a wok in cooking oil. To stir-fry, you first heat the wok to a high temperature, then add the cooking oil and broccoli. Stir often, frying for about 3 minutes. Remove from wok and add sesame oil and sesame seeds.

*4 mg per serving* *Serves 4*

### GREEN BEANS WITH DILL

Steam trimmed green beans in small amount of water with a sprig or two of fresh dill. Melt salt-free margarine or butter with lemon juice and dill weed. When green beans are slightly undercooked, drain them and pour melted lemon-dill sauce over them. Season to taste with salt substitute.

### GREEN BEANS WITH CHIVES

Steam trimmed green beans in small amount of water with garlic powder. Melt salt-free margarine or butter with chopped chives. When green beans are done but slightly undercooked drain them and pour melted chive sauce over them. Season to taste with salt substitute.

### GREEN BEANS AMANDINE

Steam trimmed green beans in small amount of water with lemon juice. Drain and add blanched almonds combined with melted salt-free margarine or butter. Season to taste with salt substitute.

*All green beans have less than 10 mg per ½ cup*

## ASPARAGUS WITH SAUCE

Steam asparagus in water with lemon juice. Serve with hot Creamed Onion Sauce or Creamed Dill Sauce (see p. 62).
*10 mg per 6 spears plus 2 tablespoons sauce*

## BAKED MASHED CARROTS

12 carrots, peeled and sliced
1½ cups water
2 tablespoons sugar or an equivalent amount of sugar substitute
3 medium apples, peeled and sliced
2 tablespoons brown sugar or an equivalent amount of sugar substitute
2 tablespoons salt-free margarine or butter
1 teaspoon cinnamon
¼ teaspoon nutmeg

Boil carrots in 1 cup of the water with sugar. When well done, drain thoroughly and mash. Simmer apples in the remaining ½ cup water with brown sugar. As soon as they soften, drain thoroughly and mash. Combine carrots, apples, 1 tablespoon of the margarine and cinnamon. Beat with fork until fluffy. Put into casserole dish. Sprinkle with nutmeg and dot top with remaining 1 tablespoon margarine. Bake at 400°F for 30 minutes or until lightly brown.
*84 mg per serving* *Serves 4*

# 6

# Eating Your Way Through the Salt-Free Day

Three meals a day and a snack here and there represent the daily diet of the salt-free life, just as they do for anyone living according to normal nutritional principles. The difference consists of watching your D.S.I. (daily sodium intake). This requires planning.

Say you're on a 1000 mgs. sodium per day diet. The best way not to exceed that amount (which admittedly isn't very much when you consider the average person in the United States eats about 5,000–15,000 mgs. per day) is to make yourself a grid and write down your meals for the entire day. (See pages 94 and 95.) At least during the early stages—once you have settled into a routine this won't be necessary. You'll be expert at estimating your D.S.I. without pen and paper. A simple way to make sure is to hold down your D.S.I. to exacting quantities where you can control it (as at home) and to avoid anything likely to contain any sodium at all where you can't. Restaurants and the homes of friends and relatives are such places, that's why we have devoted the entire next chapter to eating out.

*Breakfast:* At home it's easy. Fruit juice or fresh fruit for starters. Frozen or canned is O.K., too, but freshly squeezed is best. There are cereals, hot and cold, for sodium restricted diets, but we found regular cereals that are almost equal in sodium content and a lot cheaper. There is a low-sodium powdered milk for those on the 500 mgs. diet. Watch out for those instant brands of coffee, tea or cocoa. They're rich in sodium and have to be counted carefully. Our repertoire of eggs includes everything from soft boiled to omelets. Use that bacon flavoring called "Hickory Smoked Yeast" by Sovex, if you want to kindle old memories. Dehydrated chopped chives, fresh tomatoes and a couple of shakes of season salt substitute make an omelet taste like a delicacy. Having spent my youth in Europe, I sometimes like a fishy start. Canned tuna or salmon, preferably the low-sodium variety of "Featherweight," mixed with salt-free mayonnaise and a dash or two of lemon juice seem to do the trick. Also an excellent low-sodium line of Norwegian sardines in a variety of sauces from tomato to soy are marketed by "Featherweight," and when I don't feel like fish a piece of low-sodium hard Gouda cheese imported from the Netherlands or Cheddar from Chicago Dietetic tastes great in the morning.

I rarely feel energetic enough to start the day with breakfast at a restaurant. When I do my trusty pocket shaker of salt substitute comes in handy. Eggs of any kind present no problem, but if you really have to count your mgs., avoid fried or scrambled eggs unless you can be assured that they will be prepared with sweet butter or margarine. Fresh fruit, juice and tea make up the rest and I am sure most restaurants don't mind toasting a couple of slices of low-sodium white bread for you so bring them from home in one of those plastic sandwich bags.

*Lunch* is a different story. Since I spend most of my time working for a living and hence am not at home at this hour, I eat at my desk or entertain in a restaurant. On those happy occasions when we are at home or in our house in the country our dedication to the salt-free life can be indulged to the fullest.

For openers, a cup of chicken or beef bouillion has become something of a ritual. Lately I have added a dash or two of "Featherweight's" seasoned salt substitute and found it to be a great improvement. While I am a devotee of canned salmon and tuna fish salad on toast, Dorothy felt I would be amenable to a bit of variety and has concocted a luncheon alternative that's quick and easy to prepare and I must admit I have grown to like it. It's a toasted cheese and tomato sandwich sprinkled with one of my favorite spices, caraway seed. For the inevitable cup of soup, good old "Featherweight" comes to the rescue with a line of soups that require little doctoring and get tastier with each new shipment. They also feature a whole line of single-portion cans of lunch-type meals, from chili to ravioli, but often there are leftovers from the night before such as cold turkey or chicken or pot roast, all deliciously seasoned by Dorothy without the benefit of a grain of the white killer. Lunch, usually topped off with fresh fruit, is a feast.

Dinner remains the important meal of the day when the family meets to hold council, the dog is fed, reports are presented of the happenings of the day—dinner is serious. Usually it is the meal with the least amount of prepared food served and the greatest opportunity to meet head on the challenge of salt-free living. It is the occasion when the spice shelf turns into culinary witchcraft and the tiny sesame seed can open the doors to a world of exotic broccoli. This is also the time when man shows his true colors as a ravenous carnivore, but meat is merely toughened by salt, so there's little chance of transgression in that department. However, an enemy equally as formidable as the white killer, lurks in many clever disguises as a meat tenderizer or taste enhancer, but to me it is as deadly an enemy as its simpler forebear. Finally we reward ourselves for having so virtuously lived the salt-free life in a gastronomic celebration of dessert concoctions I have come to call our "just desserts." They range from Grand Marnier Fruit Supreme (see page 47) to frozen fruit parfaits made with ice or sherbet and a variety of fresh, frozen or canned berries that look like a rainbow at the North Pole and taste like penny candy.

Dinner, as I said, is serious.

# BREAKFAST IDEAS

**Fruit or Juice**
All fruits and fruit juices—fresh,
canned or frozen

**Breads**
LS breads
LS bread sticks
LS Grielle toast
LS crackers
Salt-free matzos
LS French toast (see p. 000)

**Spreads & Sweeteners**
Salt-free margarine
Salt-free butter
Jams and jellies
Marmalade
Apple spread
Honey
Brown sugar
White sugar
Sugar substitute

**Beverages**
Coffee
Tea
Postum
Sanka
LS* Milk

**Cereals—Dry**
LS Cornflakes
LS Corn, Puffed
LS Millet, Puffed
LS Pernola
LS Rice Krispies
LS Rice, Puffed
Rice, Puffed
LS Wheat, Puffed
Wheat, Puffed
Wheat, Shredded (spoon-sized)
Wheat, Shredded (biscuit)

**Cereals—Hot**
(Prepared without salt)
Cream of Rice
Cream of Wheat
Farina
Maltex
Malt-O-Meal
Oatmeal
Pettijohn's Wheat
Ralston
Wheatena

**Eggs**
Soft boiled
Poached
Hard boiled
Scrambled
Fried
Omelets (see p. 48)

**Cheeses**
LS Cheddar cheese
LS Colby cheese
LS Cottage cheese
LS Gouda cheese
LS Jack cheese
LS Muenster cheese
Grilled cheese (see p. 51)

**Fish**
LS Mackerel (canned)
LS Salmon (canned)
LS Sardines (canned)
LS Tuna (canned)

## SAMPLE BREAKFAST MENUS*

### I

| | PORTION | SODIUM |
|---|---|---|
| Fresh orange juice | 4 oz | 1 mg |
| Cream of Rice with cinnamon & brown sugar | ¾ cup | 10 mg |
| LS milk | ½ cup | 3 mg |
| LS bread (toast) | 2 slices | 8 mg |
| Salt-free margarine | 1 tablespoon | 1 mg |
| Apple butter | 2 tablespoons | 1 mg |
| Coffee or tea with LS milk and sweetener | 1 cup | 7 mg |
| | | 31 mg |

### II

| | PORTION | SODIUM |
|---|---|---|
| Grapefruit | ½ medium | 1 mg |
| Bacon Flavored Western Omelet (see p. 48) | 1 serving | 60 mg |
| LS bread | 2 slices | 8 mg |
| Tomato | 3 slices | 1 mg |
| Salt-free margarine | 1 tablespoon | 1 mg |
| Marmalade | 1 tablespoon | 3 mg |
| Coffee or Tea with LS milk and sugar | 1 cup | 4 mg |
| | | 78 mg |

### III

| | PORTION | SODIUM |
|---|---|---|
| Pineapple juice | 4 oz | 1 mg |
| Banana | 1 medium | 2 mg |
| Shredded wheat | 2 biscuits | 1 mg |
| LS milk | ½ cup | 3 mg |
| Salt-free matzo | 1 square | 1 mg |
| Salt-free margarine | 1 tablespoon | 1 mg |
| LS Gouda cheese | 1 oz | 12 mg |
| Coffee or tea (black) | 1 cup | 3 mg |
| | | 24 mg |

### IV

| | PORTION | SODIUM |
|---|---|---|
| Cantaloupe | ¼ melon | 12 mg |
| LS French toast (see p. 48) | 2 slices | 66 mg |
| Salt-free margarine | 1 tablespoon | 1 mg |
| Honey | 2 tablespoons | 2 mg |
| Sanka with LS milk and sweetener | 1 cup | 6 mg |
| | | 87 mg |

### V

| | PORTION | SODIUM |
|---|---|---|
| Orange and grapefruit sections | ½ cup | 1 mg |
| Sardines | 1 oz | 16 mg |
| Grilled cheese and tomato (see p. 51) | 1 slice | 13 mg |
| Coffee with LS milk, sugar and cinnamon | 1 cup | 4 mg |
| | | 34 mg |

### VI

| | PORTION | SODIUM |
|---|---|---|
| Baked apple | 1 medium | 1 mg |
| Poached egg on LS toast | 1 slice | 63 mg |
| Prune Pastry cookie (LS) | 2 cookies | 6 mg |
| Tea with lemon and sugar | 1 cup | 3 mg |
| | | 73 mg |

• Amount of sodium is based on specific brands. Be sure to check amount of sodium in the brand being used when figuring DSI (Daily Sodium Intake).

# LUNCHEON IDEAS

**Fruit or Juice**
All fresh, canned or frozen fruits
and fruit juices
LS canned tomato juice

**Soups**
LS canned soups
LS bouillon cubes
Salt-free borscht
Peter's Quick Soup (see p. 64)
Dorothy's Chicken Soup (see p. 65)

**Breads**
LS breads
LS bread sticks
LS Grielle toast
LS crackers
Salt-free matzos

**Side Dishes**
Cucumber Salad (see p. 59)
Pickled Beet Salad (see p. 60)
Coleslaw (see p. 59)
Salad greens
Lettuce hearts

**Salad Plates**
Chef Salad (see p. 57)
Fruit salad with orange ice
LS cottage cheese with sour
cream and raw vegetables
LS cottage cheese with
sour cream and fruit
Tuna Salad Plate (see p. 61)
Chicken Delight (see p. 58)
Salmon Salad Plate (see p. 58)
Egg Salad Plate (see p. 60)
Chilled LS gefilte fish
LS canned mackerel
LS canned sardines

**Hot Dishes**
All prepared meat, poultry,
fish and vegetables
(See DINNER IDEAS)
LS canned beef ravioli
LS canned beef stew
LS canned chicken stew
LS canned chili
LS canned stuffed dumplings
LS canned lamb stew

**Sandwiches**
All prepared on LS bread with
LS dressings
All meats, fish and poultry prepared
without salt
LS or salt-free peanut butter with
jelly, honey or fruit
LS canned sardines
LS canned mackerel
Cold roast beef
Cold sliced London broil
Cold sliced pot roast
Cold sliced chicken
Cold sliced turkey
Chicken Delight (see p. 58)
Tuna Salad Spread (see p. 61)
Salmon Salad Spread (see p. 60)
Egg Salad Spread (see p. 60)
Grilled Cheese (see p. 51)

**Desserts**
All fresh, canned or frozen fruits
LS gelatins
LS puddings
LS cakes and cookies

**Salad Dressings**

All LS specially prepared bottled dressings
Oil, vinegar, spices, herbs and other seasonings
Russian Dressing (see p. 63)

LS canned spaghetti with meat balls
LS canned Spanish rice
Spaghetti with garlic and salt-free butter
Spaghetti with LS tomato sauce
Noodles with salt-free butter
Tuna-Noodle Casserole (see p. 55)
Omelets (see p. 48)

Orange ice
Orange sherbet

**Beverages**

Coffee
Tea
Sanka
Postum
LS milk
Coca cola
Pepsi cola
No-Cal club soda
Schweppes ginger ale
Beer
Wine

## SAMPLE LUNCH MENUS

### I

| | PORTION | SODIUM |
|---|---|---|
| Canned vegetable soup | 1 cup | 19 mg |
| Sliced turkey sandwich (LS bread, lettuce and LS mayonnaise) | 1 | 64 mg |
| LS kosher dill pickle | 1 oz | 5 mg |
| Coca cola | 8 oz | 1 mg |
| Fresh pear | 1 medium | 4 mg |
| | | 93 mg |

### II

| | PORTION | SODIUM |
|---|---|---|
| Chef Salad (see p. 57) | 1 serving | 69 mg |
| LS Russian dressing (see p. 63) | 1 tablespoon | 5 mg |
| LS Grielle toast | 2 slices | 6 mg |
| Salt-free margarine | 1 tablespoon | 1 mg |
| Baked apple | 1 medium | 1 mg |
| Coffee with LS milk and sweetener | 1 cup | 7 mg |
| | | 89 mg |

### III

| | PORTION | SODIUM |
|---|---|---|
| LS cold borscht with sour cream (1 tablespoon) | 1 cup | 49 mg |
| Tunafish sandwich (see p. 61) | 1 | 38 mg |
| Cucumber salad (see p. 59) | 1 serving | 5 mg |
| Coffee (black) | 1 cup | 3 mg |
| Lemon wafer | 2 wafers | 12 mg |
| | | 107 mg |

### IV

| | PORTION | SODIUM |
|---|---|---|
| Grapefruit | ½ medium | 1 mg |
| LS peanut butter and jelly sandwich | 1 | 27 mg |
| Ice tea with sweetener | 8 oz | 3 mg |
| Orange ice | 1 serving | tr |
| | | 31 mg |

### V

| | PORTION | SODIUM |
|---|---|---|
| Peter's Quick Soup (see p. 64) | 1 cup | 36 mg |
| LS canned chili with 1 tablespoon chopped onions | 1 serving | 51 mg |
| Rice | ½ cup | 2 mg |
| Coleslaw (see p. 59) | 1 serving | 38 mg |
| LS crackers | 4 | 4 mg |
| Fresh fruit cup | 1 cup | 3 mg |
| Tea with lemon | 1 cup | 3 mg |
| | | 137 mg |

### VI

| | PORTION | SODIUM |
|---|---|---|
| LS Cream of mushroom soup canned (add herbs, etc.) | ½ cup | 30 mg |
| Grilled cheese sandwich (see p. 51) | 1 slice | 13 mg |
| Sanka with LS milk and sugar | 1 cup | 3 mg |
| LS gelatin with added fruit | 1 serving | 6 mg |
| | | 52 mg |

# DINNER IDEAS

**Appetizers**
All fresh, canned or frozen fruits and fruit juices
LS canned tomato juice
Salt-free gefilte fish
LS sardines
LS mackerel
Eggs à la Russe (see p. 51)
Deviled Eggs (see p. 51)
Fresh Raw Vegetables with LS Dip (see p. 52)

**Soups**
LS canned soups
LS bouillon cubes
Salt-free borscht
Homemade salt-free soup (see p. 65)

**Breads**
LS breads
LS bread sticks
LS Grielle toast
LS crackers
Salt-free matzos

**Salads**
Cucumber Salad (see p. 59)

**Entrees**
All meats prepared with herbs, spices and seasonings other than salt
Some examples:
Broiled steak with garlic and pepper
Roast beef with garlic and pepper
Pot Roast (see p. 53)
Beef Stew Burgundy (see p. 54)
London broil with garlic and paprika
Broiled liver and onions
Broiled hamburger with chopped onions and pepper
Broiled lamb chops with paprika
Roast leg of lamb with garlic cloves
Baked Pork Chops with Carrots and Pineapple (see p. 53)

All poultry prepared with herbs, spices and seasonings other than salt
Some examples:
Broiled chicken with garlic and paprika
Roast chicken with poultry seasoning and paprika
Potted Chicken

**Vegetables**
All vegetables prepared with herbs, spices and seasonings other than salt
Some examples:
Corn on the cob with melted salt-free butter and lemon juice
Baked potato with sour cream and chives
Baked sweet potato with salt-free butter and brown sugar
Baked Mashed Carrots (see p. 67)
Green Beans Amandine (see p. 66)
Green Beans with Dill (see p. 66)
Green Beans with Chives (see p. 66)
Asparagus with Sauce (see p. 67)
Broccoli with Sesame (see p. 66)

**Pastas and Rice**
Spaghetti with garlic and butter
Spaghetti with LS tomato sauce
Noodles with salt-free butter
Tuna-Noodle Casserole (see p. 55)
LS Spanish rice (canned)

**Desserts**
All fresh, frozen or canned fruits

Pickled Beet Salad (see p. 60)
Mandarin Orange Salad (see p. 58)
Coleslaw (see p. 59)
Salad greens
Tossed salad (tomato, cucumber, lettuce, green pepper and radishes)
Lettuce hearts

**Salad Dressings**
All LS specially prepared bottled dressings
Oil, vinegar, spices, herbs and other seasonings
Russian Dressing (see p. 63)

Chicken à l'Orange (see p. 56)
Roast turkey with garlic, pepper and paprika

All fish prepared with herbs, spices and seasonings other than salt
Some examples:
Halibut Baked with Dill Sauce (see p. 49)
Baked Red Snapper (see p. 50)
Curried Shrimp (see p. 50)
Shrimp Scampi (see p. 50)

LS gelatins
LS puddings
LS cakes and cookies
Orange ice
Orange sherbet
Grand Marnier Fruit Supreme (see p. 47)
Crème de Menthe Pears (see p. 47)
Applesauce

**Beverages**
Coffee
Tea
Sanka
Postum
LS milk
Coca cola
Pepsi cola
No-Cal club soda
Schweppes ginger ale
Beer
Wine

## SAMPLE DINNER MENUS

### I

| | PORTION | SODIUM |
|---|---|---|
| Deviled Eggs | ½ egg | 32 mg |
| Roast chicken (white meat) | 4 oz | 75 mg |
| Baked Mashed Carrots (see p. 67) | 1 serving | 84 mg |
| Green Beans with Chives (see p. 66) | ½ cup | 5 mg |
| Tossed salad | ½ cup | 5 mg |
| Oil and vinegar dressing | 2 tablespoons | 1 mg |
| LS bread sticks | 3 sticks | 15 mg |
| LS gelatin with fruit cocktail | 1 serving | 6 mg |
| Black coffee | 1 cup | 3 mg |
| | | 226 mg |

### II

| | PORTION | SODIUM |
|---|---|---|
| Grapefruit | ½ medium | 1 mg |
| Pot Roast (see p. 53) | 4 oz | 65 mg |
| Rice with salt-free margarine and almonds | ½ cup | 1 mg |
| Fresh green peas | ½ cup | 1 mg |
| Coleslaw (see p. 59) | 1 serving | 38 mg |
| Salt-free matzo | 1 square | 10 mg |
| Orange sherbet | 1 serving | 10 mg |
| LS cookies | 2 cookies | 10 mg |
| Ice tea (instant low-calorie diet mix) | 8 oz | 15 mg |
| | | 151 mg |

### III

| | PORTION | SODIUM |
|---|---|---|
| Salt-free gefilte fish | 1 piece | 3 mg |
| Salt-free homemade chicken soup (with rice) and chicken with vegetables from the soup | 1 serving | 150 mg |
| Applesauce | ½ cup | 2 mg |
| LS crackers | 6 crackers | 6 mg |
| Sanka with LS milk and sweetener | 1 cup | 6 mg |
| | | 167 mg |

### IV

| | PORTION | SODIUM |
|---|---|---|
| Creamed Tomato Soup (see p. 64) | 1 serving | 39 mg |
| Baked Red Snapper (see p. 50) | 1 serving | 215 mg |
| Broccoli with Sesame (see p. 66) | 1 serving | 4 mg |
| Boiled potato with parsley and salt-free margarine | 1 small | 4 mg |
| Pickled Beet Salad (see p. 60) | 1 serving | 20 mg |
| LS Grielle toast | 2 slices | 3 mg |
| Salt-free margarine | 1 tablespoon | 1 mg |
| Grand Marnier Fruit Supreme (see p. 47) | 1 serving | 7 mg |
| | | 293 mg |

## V

| | PORTION | SODIUM |
|---|---|---|
| Orange and grapefruit sections | ½ cup | 1 mg |
| Broiled lamb chops | 2 medium | 75 mg |
| Baked sweet potato | 1 small | 12 mg |
| Asparagus with Sauce (see p. 67) | 1 serving | 10 mg |
| Cucumber Salad (see p. 59) | 1 serving | 5 mg |
| LS bread | 1 slice | 4 mg |
| Salt-free margarine | 1 tablespoon | 1 mg |
| Tea with lemon and sweetener | 1 cup | 6 mg |
| LS cake | 1 slice | 2 mg |
| | | 116 mg |

## VI

| | PORTION | SODIUM |
|---|---|---|
| Fresh raw vegetables with LS Dip (see p. 52) | 1 serving | 31 mg |
| Broiled steak with garlic and pepper | 8 oz raw | 50 mg |
| Baked potato | 1 small | 4 mg |
| Broiled tomato | 1 small | 3 mg |
| Sour cream with chives | 1 oz | 13 mg |
| Crème de Menthe Pears (see p. 47) | 1 serving | 5 mg |
| Black coffee | 1 cup | 3 mg |
| | | 109 mg |

# 7

# The Low-Sodium High Life

New York City boasts restaurants for every occasion, mood or ethnic specialty. As yet it does not have a single restaurant that specializes in low-sodium cuisine, and we imagine that goes for the rest of the country as well. My job and our social life call for eating out a great deal and I've found the problem of staying on my low-sodium diet taxing but not insurmountable. So please don't think your business or social life has to be altered drastically, or that you must violate your diet every time you are eating out, just because you have to be on a salt-restricted diet. Just use some common sense, plan your salt intake for an entire day, learn what goes into preparing restaurant food and ask, ask, ask. Let me be more specific. Stay away from hors d'oeuvres you know are highly salted. The bread and butter served contains a lot of salt. A drink before and wine or beer during the meal will not seriously jeopardize your D.S.I. Orange juice gives the edge to Screwdrivers over Bloody Marys. A scotch is O.K. (because, hopefully, you'll be drinking small quantities). If you're a nondrinker, club soda has a lot more sodium in it than ginger ale, root beer or coke. Diet soft drinks contain a lot more sodium than regular ones. Our charts on beverages will help you keep a fairly accurate count.

Zero in on freshly cooked food and have the person waiting on you tell the chef to skip the salt. Broiled meat, poultry or fish are my standard entrées. Salad without dressing. I mix my own: oil and vinegar, two or three turns on the pepper mill, juice from half a lemon. Vegetables are a bit tricky because some of them contain a lot of sodium. Before going out consult our charts (spinach and carrots, for instance, are high in sodium to begin with). Avoid gravies and sauces and such obviously salty foods as sausages (including frankfurters), ham, spareribs, pork, corned beef, pastrami, pickles and all manner of smoked meat. Chinese restaurants are out of bounds; MSG, which stands for monosodium glutamate, is strictly verboten. That New York specialty, the kosher delicatessen, is also off limits. Some dairy restaurants cook without salt especially if you ask them to. Certain health food restaurants offer salt-free items on their menu but you have to clarify what they mean by what they advertise. At this writing, low-sodium diets are not yet widely understood, a situation that appears to improve with each month. If you make a mistake once in awhile or can't avoid eating something you know contains a lot of sodium, chances are you won't die from it, but don't ignore it. It pays to be pedantic about your daily salt intake and that's what I mean by planning your D.S.I. When you slip like that be extra careful and precise about the rest of the day and a day or two afterward. Planning your D.S.I. is especially important if you eat out as often as we do. When I know that we have a date for dinner at a restaurant or someone's home I am especially careful all day and since I often have business lunches as well, I try to keep track of the "unavoidables."

When I spend the lunch hour in my office, I fix myself a tray. I have a choice of salt-free canned salmon or tuna, white fresh sliced turkey meat or roast beef on tasty zwieback-type toast imported from France, called "Grielle." (I keep an insulated bagful in my desk because they keep beautifully.) Usually I precede this with a cup of bouillon (see page 69).

Invitations to friends' houses present no problem. If they're good friends we call up and brief them, if they're just new acquaintances I discreetly inform them about my problem and try to avoid their saltier creations without affecting martyrdom.

As I spend a lot of time on airplanes and out of town, I carry a salt-free kit which contains some essentials that are hard to find when you are in a strange town or 30,000 feet up in the air: salt substitute, seasoned and unseasoned; some seasonings like dill weed, curry, mustard and garlic powder, bouillon cubes and a bagful of "Grielle."

Most domestic and international airlines offer salt-free meals if you ask for them in advance. Your travel agent can do it for you or the airline's reservations department will order it for you. The chef of any cruise line will meet the challenge easily if you know what to ask for. You may encounter some difficulties in resort hotels, which pride themselves on their rich and diverse cuisine, but at one of the largest resorts in upstate New York we had no trouble and their freshly baked salt-free bread tasted delicious.

So, all in all, the outside world is not as inhospitable to those of us on a sodium-restricted diet as you might think at first. Remember the days when it was hard to find a sugar substitute in most restaurants and you had to carry your own if you wanted to be sure? The day is not far off when you won't have to carry your own salt substitute either and when many restaurants will offer low-sodium versions of their specialties. And who knows, an enterprising restaurateur might even think it worthwhile to open the first low-sodium restaurant in town. We are pleased to report that a New York restaurant by the charming name of "Greener Pastures" meets almost all the requirements of the salt-free dieter.

# 8

# Low-Sodium Dieting Without Tears (they're salty!)

Dr. Weinberg marshaled some pretty convincing facts and figures on why we should limit our sodium intake. Dorothy and I have tried to tell you how she helped me do it. The time has come to deal with the most common problem of any diet but especially the low-sodium one: *Will power*. How do you stick for long periods of time, for life perhaps, to a diet that on first reading appears to deprive you of the pleasure of eating, the sex appeal of food so to speak?

Finding tasty substitutes is one way. Having a caring and sympathetic teammate to help you over the rough spots is another. A third is Dorothy's concept of getting yourself involved in the preparation and exploration of low-sodium food. Finally, your bathroom scale and the blood pressure gauge in your doctor's office will tell you how well you're doing and nothing succeeds like success. The less sodium you consume, the less liquid your body will retain with a commensurate loss of weight and pressure. If you cheat, sneaking salty items when nobody's looking, it will soon show up on those two telltale gauges.

When that happens don't allow guilt and remorse to take over. Whatever you do, don't say to yourself: "The Hell with it! Might as well go all the way. . . ." Realize that you've come to a crisis point but that nothing is lost, yet. Tomorrow is another day for getting back to your diet. Today is for realizing that the flesh is weak and that salt can kill you.

That's what I do whenever a windowful of sausages sing their siren song for me and I break down and eat a few slices of salami, or some smoked salmon swims into my shopping bag. It also means being extra careful for the next few days in watching my D.S.I.

Don't say, "This can't happen to *me*." I haven't yet met anyone who can stay on a diet without breaking it at least once in awhile, no matter what it's for. If you're dieting for weight loss, all that may mean is that the hard work of weeks, and perhaps months, goes out the window and you have to start all over again. However, when you are on a low-sodium diet because you suffer from high blood pressure, the effects of breaking it can do incalculable harm to your system as Dr. Weinberg describes it so frighteningly elsewhere in this book. If, on the other hand, you believe in the curative effects of living salt free, you will learn to control this urge. It will help to set yourself a short-term goal of salt-free living to get over that trying period. If you can last a week or two salt free, you have licked the problem and can go on again for a long period of time.

So, when that wild craving for a salami sandwich hits you, watch out! Or better still psych yourself up against it. Don't put yourself into a situation where temptation is easily succumbed to. Like eating at a restaurant where it will be difficult or impossible to get a meal that's low in sodium content. Always have reserves of the salt-free versions of food you like to eat regularly in your kitchen. I love bread and hardly eat anything without it. I always have two or three loaves of special low-sodium bread in the freezer in the city as well as in the country, so I don't start in on the old stuff because we ran out. We do the same with low-sodium soups. It's a good principle to follow generally, since you can't shop for salt-free or low-sodium food as easily as you can for ordinary food. Not every store in your neighborhood carries a complete line of these dietetic products and you never want to have the excuse that you are breaking your diet because you ran out of a certain item and had to have its salty version "just this once." Believe me, it won't work. You'll again start comparing the two and realize something you almost managed to forget; how much more appetizing the salty version of anything tastes to our palate, accustomed as it has been in most cases, for the better part of our life, to salt consumption.

Another helpful defense against those periodic cravings for salted "no-nos" is to snack a little more often than usual. A salt-free piece of cheese with a pear or apple, roasted salt-free nuts (by Bazzini) or roasted salt-free soybeans (by Soy Town) mixed with raisins and Rice Krispies can do a lot to stop you from feeling sorry for yourself and giving in to a childish need for the bad stuff. Whenever I'm in trouble, two seasonings, particularly close to their salty versions, help me get back on the track: Whenever possible I use large amounts of low-sodium French mustard (by Jarret International of Brooklyn, N.Y.) and low-sodium dill pickles by our trusty friends at "Featherweight." Their product manager tells us they're working on a whole line of new things like that! Hope they come out with a low-sodium horseradish soon that will add some bite to "Mother's" salt-free gefilte fish!

Having a friend like Dorothy helps a lot. I tell her when I feel trouble coming on (like the night I was having a nightmare of being locked into a delicatessen and went crazy from the smell of corned beef and pastrami). When that happens, she goes into action with an array of new inventions. Between all the sampling and experimenting my head gets back in the right frame and since the palate is part of the head that does too.

The time may come when your doctor tells you that you may increase your D.S.I. to something in the neighborhood of 1,000 mgs. Obviously you are ready for a salt-binge. Take it easy and proceed with caution. You may recall what Dr. Weinberg said about the potentially deleterious effects of sodium chloride on perfectly normal, healthy people. The charts at the end of this book will help you stay within the limits of what your doctor considers a reasonable amount of the white stuff. Avoid like poison anything that sounds as if it weren't really salt, like "Light Salt" or trendy natural like "Sea Salt." It's salt by any other name.

Don't go back to using a shaker on anything. Keep a respectable distance from highly salted foods, like corned beef, pastrami, soups and bread, pretzels, salted nuts, pickles, Chinese food cooked with MSG, frankfurters, luncheon meats, ham, smoked fish or meat and, alas, every kind of wurst from liver to bologna. If you never touch them again, chances are you will be eating more than twice the amount of sodium your body needs just in your regular daily diet.

# Dorothy's Charts

# 9
# Charts

These charts provide a single source of information for all food products whether low-sodium, dietetic or regular. This will best serve to educate you about the sodium content of what you eat normally. On many occasions, while writing this book, I was amazed to discover how much sodium there was in a particular food item that did not taste "salty" at all to me.

These charts will also be useful in helping you to reduce your daily sodium intake. Very often when a person is put on a low-sodium diet, he is given a daily menu plan. For some people this works. If they are successful in altering their diet this way, they are not only reducing their daily sodium intake but are also forming better eating habits in general. However, some people find it difficult to change both their style of eating and the taste of food simultaneously. To help you devise a salt-free version of your present diet, we suggest that you use the charts in the following way.

1. Make a list of all the food you eat during the course of a normal day.
2. Look up the sodium value of each item.
3. Be as accurate as possible about the quantity of each item you eat.
4. If salt is added in the cooking normally, estimating becomes difficult. Measure its canned equivalent.
5. Compare what you ate with what your D.S.I. goal is (daily sodium intake goal).

| —1— Make a list of all of the foods that you eat in a day. (Typical diet for Peter before we started keeping track of DSI) | —2— Be as accurate as possible about the quantity of each item you eat. | —3— Look up sodium value of each item. You will find them listed under separate categories. (For example, milk is listed under dairy products; mustard under seasonings—condiments; etc.) |
|---|---|---|
| **Breakfast** | **Portion** | **Amount of sodium (mg)** |
| Orange Drink | 6 Oz | 58 |
| All Bran Cereal | ½ Cup | 370 |
| Milk | ½ Cup | 64 |
| Whole Wheat Toast | 2 Slices | 242 |
| Margarine | 1 TBSP | 138 |
| Coffee | 1 Cup | 3 |
| Milk | 1 TBSP | 8 |
| Sweet 'N Low | 1 Package | 3 |
| | | 886 mgs Total—Breakfast |
| **Lunch** | | |
| Chicken Vegetable Soup | 1 Cup | 1326 |
| Bologna | 3 Slices | 1120 |
| Rye Bread | 2 Slices | 256 |
| Mustard | 1 Tsp | 65 |
| Dill Pickle | ½ Large | 714 |
| Black Cherry TAB | 8 Oz | 63 |
| | | 3544 mgs Total—Lunch |
| **Cocktails** | | |
| Bloody Mary | 8 Oz | 400 |
| Pretzels, Salted | 10 | 1200 |
| | | 1600 mgs Total—Cocktails |
| **Dinner** | | |
| Shrimps | 4 Oz | 160 |
| Tomato Sauce | ½ Cup | 324 |
| Onion Soup | 1 Cup | 1304 |
| Steak | 8 Oz (raw) | 50 |
| Canned Asparagus | 6 Spears | 271 |
| Lettuce | ¼ Head | 12 |
| Italian Dressing | 2 TBSP | 586 |
| Apple Pie | 1/6 pie | 482 |
| Swiss Cheese | 1 Oz | 199 |
| Coffee, Black | 1 Cup | 3 |
| | | 3391 mgs Total—Dinner |

**Peter's DSI (DAILY SODIUM INTAKE) adds up to 9,421 mgs—shockingly high, especially when you consider that he was not eating excessively nor was he adding any salt from a salt shaker!!!**

—4—

**Replace high sodium items (packaged foods) with fresh food or LS (Low Sodium) dietetic substitutes.**

| Breakfast | Portion | Amount of sodium (mg) |
|---|---|---|
| Orange Juice—fresh | 4 Oz | 1 |
| Shredded Wheat | 2 Biscuits | 1 |
| Milk—LS | ½ Cup | 3 |
| White Toast—LS | 2 Slices | 8 |
| Salt Free Margarine | 1 TBSP | 1 |
| Coffee | 1 Cup | 3 |
| Milk—LS | 1 TBSP | TR |
| ZERO-CAL (sweetener) | 1 Package | 0 |
| | | 17 mgs Total—Breakfast |
| **Lunch** | | |
| Chicken Bouillon*—LS | 2 Cubes | 21 |
| Sliced Turkey | 2 Oz | 40 |
| Mayonnaise—LS | 1 TBSP | 5 |
| White Bread—LS | 2 Slices | 8 |
| Pickles—LS | 1 Oz | 5 |
| Iced Tea | 8 Oz | 3 |
| Apple, raw | 1 medium | 1 |
| | | 83 mgs Total—Lunch |
| **Cocktails** | | |
| Screwdriver | 8 Oz | 2 |
| Salt-free mixed nuts | 24 | 4 |
| | | 6 mgs Total—Cocktail |
| **Dinner** | | |
| Shrimp | 4 Oz | 160 |
| Sauce**—LS | 2 Oz | 34 |
| Steak | 8 Oz (raw) | 50 |
| Fresh Asparagus | ½ Cup | 0.8 |
| Baked Potato | 1 Small | 4 |
| Salt-free Margarine | 1 TBSP | 1 |
| Sour Cream | 1 TBSP | 13 |
| Lettuce | ¼ Head | 12 |
| Oil, Vinegar, Spices | 2 TBSP | 0.4 |
| Fresh Fruit Cup | 1 Cup | 2 |
| Cheddar Cheese—LS | 1 Oz | 5 |
| Coffee, Black | 1 Cup | 3 |
| | | 285.2 mgs Total—Dinner |

**The DSI as a result of the substitutions made is only 391 mgs—a remarkable reduction of Sodium Intake without a change in the style of eating. LS items used are Milk, Bread, Bouillon, Mayonnaise, Pickles, Sauce and Cheese.**

* Peter's Soup as described on page 64.

** Use Spaghetti Sauce LS with added spices.

6. Replace high-sodium items (packaged foods) with fresh food or low-sodium dietetic substitutes.
7. Replace the salt which you would normally add in cooking with spices and herbs. (See chapter 4).

### How to read these charts

All calculations have been expressed to the nearest whole number. Values less than one are expressed to the nearest tenth and values less than 0.1 are expressed as a trace.

Symbols used:
- DSI—Daily Sodium Intake
- tr—trace
- <—less than
- tsp—teaspoon
- g—gram
- LS—Low Sodium
- tbsp—tablespoon
- oz—ounce
- pkg—package
- lg—large
- aver.—average
- rnd.—round
- lb—pound

The low-sodium charts contain only dietetic foods manufactured specifically for low-sodium diets. However, many foods that are also low in sodium are listed in the regular charts.

Where available, the calorie, potassium, carbohydrate and fat content of all of the foods have been included to help those on other diets in addition to low sodium.

In the section on meats, those listed as cooked give the nutritional values after cooking. However, the portion described as raw means how much it weighed before cooking.

We have listed several brands of low-sodium substitutes for individual taste preference and because not all brands are available at every store. If your local market does not carry a particular item mentioned by us, you'll find a list of distributors at the end of these charts. It will help you locate any product we mention and then some! Keep looking and asking where you shop. New items come on the market every day and by asking your store manager you not only find what you need but you also raise his low-sodium consciousness by several notches.

Many sources, including some original testing, have been used to compile these charts. Wherever we use a brand name, the source for that information is either directly from the company itself or from their printed label. Because of the variance in soil and water in different parts of the country, there is a natural variance in the sodium content of natural foods. We have tried to give you what we feel is an average value of content.

We thank all of the manufacturers for their cooperation.

| CATEGORY & FOOD | PORTION | SODIUM (mg) | POTASSIUM (mg) | CALORIES | CARBOHYDRATES (g) | FAT (g) |
|---|---|---|---|---|---|---|
| **Baby Foods—Cereals** | | | | | | |
| barley | 6 tbsp | 1 | | 55 | 11 | 1 |
| high protein | 6 tbsp | 1 | | 55 | 6 | 1 |
| mixed | 6 tbsp | 1 | | 55 | 11 | 1 |
| oatmeal | 6 tbsp | 1 | | 55 | 10 | 1 |
| rice | 6 tbsp | 1 | | 55 | 11 | 1 |
| **Baby Foods—Desserts** | | | | | | |
| custard puddings | 1 jar | 150 | | 125 | 25 | 2 |
| fruit puddings | 1 jar | 128 | | 100 | 22 | 1 |
| **Baby Foods—Dinners** | | | | | | |
| beef noodle | 1 jar | 163 | | 60 | 9 | 1 |
| cereal, egg yolk, bacon | 1 jar | 172 | | 95 | 9 | 5 |
| chicken noodle | 1 jar | 147 | | 60 | 10 | 1 |
| macaroni, tomatoes, meat | 1 jar | 137 | | 80 | 12 | 3 |
| split peas, vegetables, ham | 1 jar | 295 | | 80 | 11 | 2 |
| vegetables and bacon | 1 jar | 183 | | 95 | 13 | 4 |
| vegetables and beef | 1 jar | 173 | | 70 | 9 | 3 |

| | | | | | |
|---|---|---|---|---|---|
| vegetables and chicken | 1 jar | 137 | 55 | 9 | 1 |
| vegetables and ham | 1 jar | 298 | 70 | 10 | 3 |
| vegetables and lamb | 1 jar | 184 | 65 | 10 | 2 |
| vegetables and liver | 1 jar | 262 | 80 | 8 | 4 |
| vegetables and turkey | 1 jar | 157 | 60 | 11 | 1 |
| **Baby Foods—Fruits** | | | | | |
| applesauce | 1 jar | 2 | 110 | 27 | <1 |
| applesauce and apricots | 1 jar | 2 | 120 | 29 | <1 |
| apricots with tapioca | 1 jar | 42 | 110 | 26 | <1 |
| bananas with tapioca | 1 jar | 39 | 120 | 29 | <1 |
| peaches | 1 jar | 3 | 110 | 26 | <1 |
| pears | 1 jar | 3 | 90 | 23 | <1 |
| pears and pineapple | 1 jar | 3 | 95 | 23 | <1 |
| plums with tapioca | 1 jar | 47 | 140 | 35 | <1 |
| prunes with tapioca | 1 jar | 26 | 120 | 29 | <1 |
| **Baby Foods—Meats, Poultry and Eggs** | | | | | |
| beef | 1 jar | 180 | 90 | 0 | 4 |
| beef with heart | 1 jar | 149 | 85 | 1 | 4 |
| beef liver | 1 jar | 160 | 95 | 2 | 3 |
| chicken | 1 jar | 168 | 130 | <1 | 9 |

| CATEGORY & FOOD | PORTION | SODIUM (mg) | POTASSIUM (mg) | CALORIES | CARBOHYDRATES (g) | FAT (g) |
|---|---|---|---|---|---|---|
| egg yolks | 1 jar | 165 | | 190 | 0 | 17 |
| egg yolks and ham | 1 jar | 312 | | 185 | 0 | 16 |
| ham | 1 jar | 200 | | 115 | 1 | 6 |
| lamb | 1 jar | 164 | | 95 | 0 | 4 |
| pork | 1 jar | 218 | | 110 | 0 | 6 |
| turkey | 1 jar | 180 | | 130 | <1 | 8 |
| veal | 1 jar | 177 | | 90 | 0 | 4 |
| **Baby Foods—Vegetables** | | | | | | |
| beets | 1 jar | 205 | | 50 | 10 | <1 |
| carrots | 1 jar | 156 | | 40 | 8 | <1 |
| corn, creamed | 1 jar | 129 | | 85 | 18 | <1 |
| garden | 1 jar | 142 | | 40 | 7 | <1 |
| green beans | 1 jar | 146 | | 40 | 7 | <1 |
| mixed | 1 jar | 218 | | 50 | 11 | <1 |
| peas | 1 jar | 129 | | 55 | 9 | <1 |
| spinach, creamed | 1 jar | 150 | | 55 | 8 | 1 |
| squash | 1 jar | 129 | | 35 | 7 | <1 |
| sweet potatoes | 1 jar | 135 | | 95 | 21 | <1 |

| Baked Goods—Breads | | | | | | |
|---|---|---|---|---|---|---|
| Boston brown | 1 slice | 88 | 104 | 74 | 16 | 0.5 |
| corn bread | 2" square | 283 | 71 | 93 | 13 | 3 |
| cracked wheat | 1 slice | 122 | 31 | 60 | 12 | 0.1 |
| French or Vienna | 1 slice | 116 | 18 | 58 | 11 | 0.6 |
| Italian | 1 slice | 117 | 15 | 55 | 11 | 0.2 |
| pumpernickle | 1 slice | 182 | 145 | 79 | 17 | 0.4 |
| raisin | 1 slice | 84 | 54 | 60 | 12 | 0.6 |
| rye | 1 slice | 128 | 33 | 56 | 12 | 0.3 |
| white | 1 slice | 117 | 20 | 62 | 12 | 0.7 |
| whole wheat | 1 slice | 121 | 63 | 56 | 11 | 0.7 |

| Baked Goods—Breads—Especially Prepared for Low-Sodium Diets | | | | | | |
|---|---|---|---|---|---|---|
| Babara whole wheat bread sticks | 1 stick | 5 | | | | |
| Bloomingdale's low-sodium white bread | 1 oz | 2 | | | | |
| Bread for life | 1 slice | 4 | | | | |
| Cohen's Bakery, no-salt bread | 1 slice | 12 | | | | |
| Freihofer low-sodium bread | 1 slice | 4 | | | | |
| Grielle toast | 1 piece | 3 | | 30 | 6 | 0.4 |
| Levy's white bread | 1 slice | 2 | | 84 | 15 | 2 |
| Wuest soya protein bread | 1 slice | 4 | | | | |

| CATEGORY & FOOD | PORTION | SODIUM (mg) | POTASSIUM (mg) | CALORIES | CARBOHYDRATES (g) | FAT (g) |
|---|---|---|---|---|---|---|
| **Baked Goods—Cakes** | | | | | | |
| angel food cake | 1 aver. piece* | 127 | 40 | 121 | 27 | 0.1 |
| brownie | 2" x 2" x ¾" | 75 | 57 | 146 | 15 | 9 |
| Chocolate Pinwheels—Nabisco | 1 cake | 45 | 55 | 140 | 21 | 5 |
| cupcake, plain | 1 cake | 120 | 32 | 146 | 22 | 6 |
| devil's food cake | 2" x 3" x 2" | 132 | 63 | 165 | 23 | 8 |
| fruitcake, dark | 1 aver. piece* | 63 | 198 | 152 | 34 | 6 |
| fruitcake, light | 1 aver. piece* | 77 | 93 | 156 | 23 | 7 |
| pound cake, plain | 1 aver. piece* | 33 | 18 | 142 | 14 | 9 |
| sponge cake | 1 aver. piece* | 84 | 44 | 149 | 27 | 3 |
| white cake | 1 aver. piece* | 162 | 38 | 188 | 27 | 8 |
| yellow cake | 1 aver. piece* | 129 | 39 | 182 | 29 | 6 |
| **Baked Goods—Cake Icing** | | | | | | |
| caramel | 1 portion | 8 | 5 | 36 | 8 | 0.7 |
| chocolate | 1 portion | 6 | 20 | 38 | 7 | 1 |
| coconut | 1 portion | 12 | 17 | 36 | 8 | 0.8 |
| white | 1 portion | 5 | 2 | 38 | 8 | 0.7 |

* 1 average piece—3" x 3" x ½"

| | | | | | | |
|---|---|---|---|---|---|---|
| **Baked Goods—Cakes—Especially Prepared for Low-Sodium Diets** | | | | | | |
| cake, low-sodium—Cellu | ½" slice | 6 | | 191 | 20 | 12 |
| fruitcake, salt-free—Holland Honey | ½" slice | 2 | | 80 | 19 | 0 |
| plain cake, salt-free—Holland Honey | ½" slice | 1 | | 70 | 18 | 0 |
| **Baked Goods—Cake and Cookie Mixes, Leavenings—Especially Prepared for Low-Sodium Diets** | | | | | | |
| cake mix—Swansdown cake flour | 1 cup | 3 | | 350 | 75 | 2 |
| cake and cookie mix—Cellu | 1 slice | 15 | | 170 | 24 | 7 |
| low protein baking mix—Cellu | ½" slice | 21 | | 113 | 23 | 2 |
| yellow cake mix, low-sodium—Van Winkle | 1 slice | 10 | 183 | 171 | 26 | 7 |
| **Baked Goods—Cookies** | | | | | | |
| Almond Flavored Crescents—Nabisco | 1 cookie | 29 | 8 | 35 | 5 | 1.5 |
| Animal Crackers, Barnum—Nabisco | 1 cracker | 14 | 3 | 12 | 2 | 0.4 |
| assorted | 1-2" | 73 | 13 | 96 | 14 | 4 |
| Biscos sugar wafers—Nabisco | 1 wafer | 20 | 2 | 19 | 3 | 0.9 |
| Biscos waffle cremes—Nabisco | 1 cookie | 13 | 2 | 43 | 6 | 2 |
| Brown edge wafers—Nabisco | 1 wafer | 21 | 8 | 28 | 4 | 1 |
| Butter flavored cookies—Nabisco | 1 cookie | 25 | 7 | 23 | 4 | 0.8 |
| butter cookies | 1-2½" | 46 | 7 | 50 | 8 | 2 |
| Cameo creme sandwich—Nabisco | 1 cookie | 45 | 18 | 70 | 11 | 3 |
| Chips Ahoy, chocolate chip—Nabisco | 1 cookie | 33 | 15 | 53 | 7 | 2 |

| CATEGORY & FOOD | PORTION | SODIUM (mg) | POTASSIUM (mg) | CALORIES | CARBOHYDRATES (g) | FAT (g) |
|---|---|---|---|---|---|---|
| chocolate chip | 1 cookie | 44 | 15 | 52 | 8 | 2 |
| Chocolate grahams—Nabisco | 1 cracker | 67 | 40 | 57 | 7 | 3 |
| Cinnamon sugar ring cookies—Nabisco | 1 cookie | 45 | 10 | | | |
| Cinnamon treats—Nabisco | 1 cracker | 41 | 10 | 28 | 5 | 0.5 |
| Cocoanut bars cookies—Nabisco | 1 cookie | 40 | 20 | 47 | 6 | 2 |
| cocoanut bar | 1 bar | 33 | 50 | 109 | 14 | 5 |
| Cocoanut chocolate chip—Nabisco | 1 cookie | 65 | 28 | | | |
| Cocoanut macaroon cookie—Nabisco | 1 cookie | 33 | 18 | 60 | 7 | 3 |
| Cookie break, mixed cremes—Nabisco | 1 cookie | 33 | 8 | | | |
| Cowboys and Indians cookies—Nabisco | 1 cookie | 12 | 2 | 10 | 2 | 0.3 |
| Creme wafer sticks—Nabisco | 1 stick | 13 | 13 | 50 | 6 | 3 |
| Famous chocolate wafers—Nabisco | 1 wafer | 48 | 19 | 28 | 5 | 0.8 |
| Fancy dip grahams—Nabisco | 1 piece | 40 | 28 | 65 | 9 | 3 |
| Fig Newton cakes—Nabisco | 1 cake | 63 | 38 | 55 | 12 | 1 |
| Ginger Snaps | 1 small | 23 | 18 | 17 | 3 | 0.4 |
| Graham Crackers—Nabisco | 1 cracker | 45 | 175 | 30 | 7 | 0.8 |
| Honey Maid graham crackers—Nabisco | 1 cracker | 48 | 10 | 30 | 6 | 0.8 |
| Lorna Doone shortbread—Nabisco | 1 cookie | 38 | 9 | 40 | 5 | 2 |
| Macaroons | 1 medium | 5 | 65 | 67 | 9 | 3 |
| Mallomars chocolate cakes—Nabisco | 1 cake | 23 | 23 | 55 | 9 | 2 |

| | | | | | | |
|---|---|---|---|---|---|---|
| marshmallow | 1 | cookie | 59 | 25 | 114 | 20 | 4 |
| Marshmallow puffs—Nabisco | 1 | cookie | 40 | 33 | 85 | 13 | 4 |
| Marshmallow sandwich—Nabisco | 1 | cookie | 20 | 6 | 33 | 6 | .8 |
| Mystic mint sandwich cookies—Nabisco | 1 | cookie | 73 | 38 | 85 | 11 | 5 |
| National arrowroot biscuit—Nabisco | 1 | biscuit | 16 | 7 | 20 | 4 | 1 |
| Nilla wafers—Nabisco | 1 | wafer | 16 | 5 | 19 | 3 | 0.6 |
| Nutter Butter, peanut butter—Nabisco | 1 | cookie | 68 | 33 | 70 | 10 | 3 |
| Oatmeal cookies—Nabisco | 1 | cookie | 73 | 18 | 75 | 12 | 3 |
| Oatmeal and raisin cookies | 1 | 3" | 23 | 52 | 63 | 10 | 2 |
| Old-fashion gingersnap—Nabisco | 1 | cookie | 46 | 49 | 30 | 6 | 0.8 |
| Oreo chocolate sandwich cookie—Nabisco | 1 | cookie | 80 | 23 | 50 | 7 | 2 |
| peanut cookie | 1 | cookie | 21 | 21 | 57 | 8 | 2 |
| Peanut creme patties—Nabisco | 1 | cookie | 21 | 19 | 35 | 4 | 2 |
| Pecan shortbread cookies—Nabisco | 1 | cookie | 45 | 13 | 80 | 9 | 5 |
| raisin cookie | 1 | cookie | 8 | 41 | 57 | 12 | 0.8 |
| Raisin fruit biscuit—Nabisco | 1 | biscuit | 35 | 75 | 55 | 12 | 0.5 |
| sandwich cookies | 1 | cookie | 68 | 5 | 69 | 10 | 3 |
| shortbread cookies | 1 | cookie | 4 | 5 | 35 | 5 | 2 |
| Social Tea biscuits—Nabisco | 1 | biscuit | 28 | 5 | 20 | 4 | 0.5 |
| Spiced wafers—Nabisco | 1 | wafer | 50 | 25 | 33 | 6 | 1 |
| sugar cookies | 1 | 3" | 64 | 15 | 89 | 14 | 3 |
| Sugar ring cookies—Nabisco | 1 | cookie | 53 | 13 | 70 | 11 | 3 |
| Sugar wafers | 1 | wafer | 11 | 4 | 27 | 4 | 1 |

| CATEGORY & FOOD | PORTION | SODIUM (mg) | POTASSIUM (mg) | CALORIES | CARBOHYDRATES (g) | FAT (g) |
|---|---|---|---|---|---|---|
| vanilla wafers | 1 wafer | 9 | 3 | 17 | 3 | 0.6 |
| Waverly wafers—Nabisco | 1 wafer | 39 | 5 | 18 | 3 | 0.8 |
| Zwieback toast—Nabisco | 1 toast | 13 | 14 | 30 | 5 | 1 |

| Baked Goods—Cookies—Especially Prepared for Low-Sodium Diets | | | | | | |
|---|---|---|---|---|---|---|
| Apple pastry—Stella D'Oro | 1 cookie | 28 | | 105 | 14 | 5 |
| Assorted filled wafers—Estee | 1 wafer | 3 | | 30 | | |
| Bittersweet wafers—Estee | 1 wafer | 3 | | 115 | | |
| Chocolate chip cookies—Estee | 1 cookie | 7 | | 30 | | |
| Duplex sandwich cookies—Estee | 1 cookie | 3 | | 50 | | |
| Fruit flavored wafers—Estee | 1 wafer | 0.6 | | | | |
| Holland filled chocolate wafers—Estee | 1 wafer | 3 | | | | |
| Holland filled wafers—Estee | 1 wafer | 0.7 | | | | |
| Lemon wafers—El Molino | 1 wafer | 6 | | | | |
| Lemon sandwich cookie—Estee | 1 cookie | 20 | | 60 | | |
| Love cookies, low-sodium—Stella D'Oro | 1 cookie | 3 | | 110 | 13 | 6 |
| Milk chocolate flavored wafers—Estee | 1 wafer | 9 | | 115 | | |
| Oatmeal raisin—Estee | 1 cookie | 2 | | 30 | | |
| Peach apricot pastry—Stella D'Oro | 1 cookie | 3 | | 110 | 14 | 6 |
| Prune pastry—Stella D'Oro | 1 cookie | 5 | | 110 | 14 | 6 |

| | | | | | | |
|---|---|---|---|---|---|---|
| Vanilla and chocolate filled wafers—Estee | 1 wafer | 3 | | | | |

**Baked Goods—Crackers**

| | | | | | | |
|---|---|---|---|---|---|---|
| American harvest snack cracker | 1 cracker | 37 | 11 | 16 | 2 | 0.8 |
| Bacon Flavored thin crackers | 1 cracker | 30 | 4 | 11 | 2 | 1 |
| Buttery flavored sesame snack crackers | 1 cracker | 21 | 3 | 17 | 2 | 0.9 |
| Cheddar 'n Chips cheese flavored thins | 1 cracker | 15 | 0.8 | 8 | 0.9 | 0.4 |
| Cheese Nips artificial flavored crackers | 1 cracker | 15 | 2 | 6 | 0.7 | 0.3 |
| Chicken In a Biskit flavored crackers | 1 cracker | 18 | 5 | 10 | 1 | 0.6 |
| Crown pilot crackers | 1 cracker | 80 | 23 | 70 | 13 | 2 |
| Dandy soup and oyster crackers | 1 cracker | 13 | 1 | 3 | 0.6 | 0.1 |
| Escort crackers | 1 cracker | 48 | 4 | 21 | 3 | 1 |
| French onion crackers | 1 cracker | 37 | 4 | 12 | 2 | 0.6 |
| Oysterettes soup and oyster crackers | 1 cracker | 8 | 1 | 3 | 0.6 | 0.1 |
| Premium crackers, unsalted tops | 1 cracker | 25 | 5 | 12 | 2 | 0.3 |
| Premium Plus, saltier saltine crackers | 1 cracker | 56 | 5 | 12 | 2 | 0.3 |
| Premium Saltine crackers | 1 cracker | 43 | 5 | 12 | 2 | 0.3 |
| Ritz crackers | 1 cracker | 32 | 4 | 17 | 2 | 0.9 |
| Ritz cheese crackers | 1 cracker | 37 | 4 | 18 | 2 | 1 |
| Sociable crackers | 1 cracker | 24 | 5 | 10 | 1 | 0.4 |
| Triangle thins crackers | 1 cracker | 21 | 4 | 8 | 1 | 0.4 |
| Triscuit wafers | 1 wafer | 34 | 16 | 20 | 3 | 0.7 |
| Uneeda biscuit, unsalted tops | 1 biscuit | 42 | 8 | 22 | 4 | 0.5 |

| CATEGORY & FOOD | PORTION | SODIUM (mg) | POTASSIUM (mg) | CALORIES | CARBOHYDRATES (g) | FAT (g) |
|---|---|---|---|---|---|---|
| Wheat thins crackers | 1 cracker | 16 | 4 | 9 | 1 | 0.4 |
| **Baked Goods—Crackers—Especially Prepared for Low-Sodium Diets** | | | | | | |
| Baron de Natural, whole wheat-froumene | 1 cracker | 2 | | 46 | | |
| Matzos, dietetic—Goodman's | 1 cracker | <3 | | 10 | 2 | 0 |
| Matzos, midgetta—Goodman's | 1 cracker | <0.3 | | | | |
| Matzos, regular, unsalted—Goodman's | 1 square | <10 | | 130 | 26 | 1 |
| Matzos, reg., round, unsalted—Goodman's | 1 round | 0.4 | | 70 | | |
| Matzos, unsalted—Manischewitz | 1 matzo | 0.6 | | | | |
| Matzos, dietetic—Streitz | 1 matzo | <10 | | 120 | 23 | 1 |
| Matzos, regular, unsalted—Streitz | 1 matzo | 2 | | | | |
| Melba toast—Cellu | 1 slice | <3 | | 15 | 3 | 0.2 |
| Melba toast, plain, unsalted—Devonshire | 1 round | 1 | | 16 | 3 | 0 |
| Melba toast, rye, unsalted, Devonshire | 1 round | 1 | | 16 | 3 | 0 |
| Melba toast, whole wheat, unsalted—Devonshire | 1 round | 1 | | 16 | 3 | 0 |
| Rice cakes, salt-free—Chico San | 1 cracker | 3 | | 26 | 6 | 0.2 |
| Rice crunch, salt-free—Ka-Me | 1 cracker | 0.5 | | | | |
| Unsalted crackers—Cellu | 1 cracker | 0.3 | | 15 | 3 | 0.4 |
| Waferettes, rice, salt-free—Hol-Grain | 1 wafer | 0.3 | | 12 | | |

| | | | | | | |
|---|---|---|---|---|---|---|
| Waferettes, whole wheat, salt-free—Hol-Grain | 1 | wafer | 0.3 | | 7 | | |
| Wafers, all grane, unsalted—Devonshire | | | | | | | |
| Wafers, rice, unsalted—Devonshire | 1 | wafer | 0.2 | | 9 | 2 | 0.1 |
| Wafers, salt-free—Venus | 1 | wafer | 1 | | 18 | 3 | 0.5 |
| Wafers, whole rice—Cellu | 1 | wafer | <3 | | 9 | 2 | 0 |
| Waldorf low-sodium crackers—Keebler | 1 | section | 1 | | | | |
| Whole rice cracker—Ryvita | 1 | cracker | 0.8 | | | | |
| **Baked Goods—Muffins** | | | | | | | |
| blueberry muffins | 1 | aver. | 253 | 46 | 112 | 17 | 4 |
| corn muffins | 1 | aver. | 216 | 61 | 141 | 22 | 5 |
| plain muffins | 1 | aver. | 176 | 50 | 118 | 17 | 4 |
| whole wheat muffins | 1 | aver. | 226 | 117 | 103 | 21 | 1 |
| **Baked Goods—Pancakes and Waffle** | | | | | | | |
| buckwheat | 1 | aver. | 209 | 110 | 90 | 11 | 4 |
| popover | 1 | aver. | 110 | 75 | 112 | 13 | 5 |
| regular | 1 | aver. | 191 | 55 | 104 | 15 | 3 |
| waffle | 1 | aver. | 356 | 109 | 209 | 28 | 7 |

| CATEGORY & FOOD | PORTION | SODIUM (mg) | POTASSIUM (mg) | CALORIES | CARBOHYDRATES (g) | FAT (g) |
|---|---|---|---|---|---|---|
| **Baked Goods—Pies** | | | | | | |
| apple pie | 1/6 pie | 482 | 128 | 410 | 61 | 18 |
| blueberry pie | 1/6 pie | 429 | 104 | 387 | 56 | 17 |
| cherry pie | 1/6 pie | 486 | 168 | 418 | 62 | 18 |
| chocolate chiffon pie | 1/6 pie | 403 | 176 | 525 | 70 | 25 |
| chocolate meringue pie | 1/6 pie | 385 | 209 | 378 | 50 | 18 |
| cocoa custard pie | 1/6 pie | 284 | 253 | 365 | 39 | 19 |
| custard pie | 1/6 pie | 430 | 205 | 327 | 35 | 17 |
| lemon chiffon pie | 1/6 pie | 279 | 87 | 335 | 47 | 14 |
| lemon meringue pie | 1/6 pie | 395 | 70 | 357 | 53 | 14 |
| mince pie | 1/6 pie | 716 | 285 | 434 | 66 | 18 |
| peach pie | 1/6 pie | 246 | | 421 | 63 | 18 |
| pecan pie | 1/6 pie | 354 | 197 | 668 | 82 | 37 |
| pineapple pie | 1/6 pie | 434 | 115 | 404 | 61 | 17 |
| pumpkin pie | 1/6 pie | 321 | 240 | 317 | 37 | 17 |
| raisin pie | 1/6 pie | 342 | 231 | 325 | 33 | 13 |
| rhubarb pie | 1/6 pie | 432 | 254 | 405 | 61 | 17 |
| sweet potato pie | 1/6 pie | 349 | 261 | 342 | 38 | 18 |

| **Baked Goods—Rolls** | | | | | | |
|---|---|---|---|---|---|---|
| biscuits | 2" biscuit | 219 | 41 | 129 | 16 | 6 |
| frankfurter rolls | 1 aver. | 205 | | 115 | 19 | 3 |
| hamburger rolls | 1 aver. | 152 | 28 | 89 | 16 | 2 |
| hard white rolls | 1 aver. | 219 | 34 | 109 | 21 | 1 |
| soft dinner rolls | 1 aver. | 90 | | 80 | 20 | 3 |
| whole wheat rolls | 1 aver. | 197 | 102 | 90 | 18 | 1 |

| **Baked Goods—Sweet Rolls and Pastries** | | | | | | |
|---|---|---|---|---|---|---|
| cinnamon raisin buns | 1 aver. | 230 | 147 | 165 | 34 | 2 |
| Danish pastry | 1 small | 128 | 39 | 148 | 16 | 8 |
| doughnuts | 1 aver. | 160 | 29 | 125 | 16 | 6 |
| Honey buns—Morton | 1 bun | 32 | | 145 | 22 | 6 |
| hot cross buns | 1 bun | 136 | 43 | 111 | 17 | 3 |
| Toaster pastry—Krazy Glazy | 1 pastry | 175 | 60 | 210 | 17 | 5 |
| Toaster pastry—Toastettes | 1 pastry | 170 | 55 | 190 | 35 | 5 |

| **Beverages—Alcoholic** | | | | | | |
|---|---|---|---|---|---|---|
| beer | 8 oz | 16 | 15 | 96 | 9 | 0 |
| gin, rum, vodka, whiskey | 1 oz | 0.3 | 0.6 | 66 | tr | 0 |
| wine—dessert | 3½ oz | 4 | 75 | 137 | 8 | 0 |

| CATEGORY & FOOD | PORTION | SODIUM (mg) | POTASSIUM (mg) | CALORIES | CARBOHYDRATES (g) | FAT (g) |
|---|---|---|---|---|---|---|
| wine—table | 3½ oz | 5 | 92 | 85 | 4 | 0 |
| **Beverages—Fruit Flavored and Fruit Juice—See Fruits** | | | | | | |
| **Beverages—Milk—See Dairy Products** | | | | | | |
| **Beverages—Other** | | | | | | |
| cocoa—instant—(½ milk) | 1 cup | 128 | | 112 | 20 | 3 |
| cocoa—instant—Alba 66 | 1 pkg | 96 | | 70 | 12 | 0 |
| coffee—brewed | 1 cup | 3 | 149 | 5 | 0.8 | 0.1 |
| coffee—instant | 1 tsp | 6 | | 4 | 1 | 0 |
| eggnog—(all milk) | 8 oz | 156 | 326 | 291 | 25 | 15 |
| Metrecal | 8 oz | 225 | | 225 | 28 | 5 |
| Postum—instant | 6 oz | 5 | 94 | 12 | 3 | 0 |
| Sanka—instant | 1 tsp | 2 | | 4 | 1 | 0 |
| Sego | 8 oz | 176 | 704 | 180 | 21 | 4 |
| Sustagen | 8 oz | 210 | 770 | 390 | 67 | 3 |
| tea | 8 oz | 3 | 25 | 2 | 0.4 | 0 |

| | | | | | | |
|---|---|---|---|---|---|---|
| tea—Instant—diet mix | 8 oz | 15 | | 5 | 1 | 0 |
| **Beverages—Soft Drinks (Carbonated)** | | | | | | |
| Birch beer—Canada Dry | 8 oz | 17 | | 100 | 26 | 0 |
| Bitter lemon—Canada Dry | 8 oz | 17 | | 100 | 26 | 0 |
| Bitter lemon—Schweppes | 8 oz | 40 | | 130 | 32 | 0 |
| Black cherry—diet—Canada Dry | 8 oz | 48 | | 2 | <1 | 2 |
| Black cherry—diet—Tab | 8 oz | 63 | | 3 | tr | 0 |
| Club soda—Canada Dry | 8 oz | 60 | | <1 | 0 | 0 |
| Club soda—Schweppes | 8 oz | 35 | | 0 | 0 | 0 |
| Coffee—diet—Canada Dry | 8 oz | 53 | | 2 | <1 | 2 |
| Cola—diet—Canada Dry | 8 oz | 11 | | 1 | <1 | 0 |
| Cola—Coca-Cola | 8 oz | 1 | 117 | 96 | 24 | 0 |
| Cola—Diet Rite | 8 oz | 39 | | <1 | <1 | 0 |
| Cola—Pepsi | 8 oz | 1 | 7 | 105 | 27 | 1 |
| Cola—diet—Pepsi | 8 oz | 32 | | 1 | 1 | 0 |
| Cream—Canada Dry | 8 oz | 17 | | 130 | 33 | 0 |
| Cream—diet—Canada Dry | 8 oz | 30 | | 1 | 1 | 0 |
| Ginger ale—Canada Dry | 8 oz | 48 | | 85 | 22 | 0 |
| Ginger ale—diet—Canada Dry | 8 oz | 20 | | 3 | 1 | 0 |
| Ginger ale—Schweppes | 8 oz | 0 | | 90 | 22 | 0 |
| Ginger ale—diet—Tab | 8 oz | 48 | | 2 | tr | 0 |
| Grape—Canada Dry | 8 oz | 18 | | 130 | 32 | 0 |

| CATEGORY & FOOD | PORTION | SODIUM (mg) | POTASSIUM (mg) | CALORIES | CARBOHYDRATES (g) | FAT (g) |
|---|---|---|---|---|---|---|
| Half and half—Canada Dry | 8 oz | 17 | | 100 | 27 | 0 |
| Lemon—diet—Canada Dry | 8 oz | 31 | | 2 | 1 | 0 |
| Orange—Canada Dry | 8 oz | 20 | | 125 | 24 | 0 |
| Orange—diet—Canada Dry | 8 oz | 20 | | 1 | 1 | 0 |
| Pink grapefruit—diet—Canada Dry | 8 oz | 17 | | 1 | 1 | 0 |
| Root beer—diet—Canada Dry | 8 oz | 16 | | 1 | 1 | 0 |
| Strawberry—diet—Canada Dry | 8 oz | 19 | | 1 | 1 | 0 |
| Tab—diet | 8 oz | 17 | | 1 | tr | 0 |
| Tonic water—Canada Dry | 8 oz | 0 | | 90 | 22 | 0 |
| Wild cherry—Canada Dry | 8 oz | 17 | | 130 | 32 | 0 |
| **Beverages—Soft Drinks (Carbonated) Especially Prepared for Low-Sodium Diets** | | | | | | |
| Club soda—No-Cal | 8 oz | 0.5 | | 0 | 0 | 0 |
| **Cereals—Dry** | | | | | | |
| Alpha Bits—Post's | 1 cup | 211 | 54 | 110 | 24 | 0.1 |
| Barley—Gerber's | 1 cup | 215 | 149 | 128 | 27 | 0.2 |
| Bran, all—Kellogg's | ½ cup | 370 | | 95 | 21 | 0.7 |
| Bran, all—Nabisco | ½ cup | 235 | 345 | 70 | 21 | 2 |
| Bran flakes, 40%—Kellogg's | ¾ cup | 340 | | 101 | 23 | 0.6 |

| | | | | | | |
|---|---|---|---|---|---|---|
| Bran flakes, 40%—Post's | ¾ cup | 314 | 169 | 113 | 25 | 1 |
| Bran, raisin—Kellogg's | ½ cup | 280 | | 73 | 17 | 0.4 |
| Bran, raisin—Post's | ½ cup | 194 | 149 | 100 | 22 | 1 |
| Cheerios—General Mills' | 1 cup | 275 | | 102 | 18 | 2 |
| Cocoa Pebbles—Post's | 1 cup | 178 | 73 | 126 | 30 | 0 |
| Corn flakes | 1 cup | 165 | 40 | 95 | 21 | 0.1 |
| Crispy Critters—Post's | 1 cup | 225 | 70 | 110 | 24 | 0 |
| Fortified oat flakes—Post's | ¾ cup | 353 | 115 | 124 | 23 | 1 |
| Fruity Pebbles—Post's | 1 cup | 182 | 47 | 126 | 30 | 0 |
| Grapenuts—Post's | ¼ cup | 174 | 75 | 100 | 23 | 0 |
| Grapenut Flakes—Post's | 1 cup | 230 | 103 | 114 | 26 | 1 |
| High protein—Gerber's | ¾ cup | 159 | 41 | 110 | 26 | 0 |
| Hi Pro—General Mills' | 1 cup | 294 | | 80 | 14 | 0.3 |
| Honey Comb—Post's | 1 cup | 176 | 31 | 83 | 19 | 0 |
| Kix—General Mills' | 1 cup | 275 | | 99 | 20 | 1 |
| Mixed cereals—Gerber's | ½ cup | 126 | 72 | 76 | 15 | 0.3 |
| Post Toasties | 1 cup | 260 | 23 | 88 | 19 | 0 |
| Rice Krinkles—Post's | 1 cup | 255 | 43 | 126 | 30 | 0 |
| Rice Krispies—Kellogg's | 1 cup | 280 | | 107 | 25 | 0.1 |
| Rice, Puffed—Quaker's | 1 cup | 0.3 | | 51 | 12 | 0.1 |
| Special K—Kellogg's | 1 cup | 193 | | 60 | 13 | 0.1 |
| Team Flakes—Nabisco | 1 cup | 250 | 65 | 110 | 24 | 1 |
| Wheaties—General Mills' | 1 cup | 392 | | 104 | 23 | 0.6 |

| CATEGORY & FOOD | PORTION | SODIUM (mg) | POTASSIUM (mg) | CALORIES | CARBOHYDRATES (g) | FAT (g) |
|---|---|---|---|---|---|---|
| Wheat, puffed—Quaker's | 1 cup | 1 | | 43 | 10 | 0.2 |
| Wheat, spoon size shredded—Nabisco | ¾ cup | 0.7 | 129 | 124 | 26 | 1 |
| Wheat, shredded—Nabisco | 1 biscuit | 0.5 | 100 | 90 | 19 | 1 |
| Wheat chex—Ralston | ½ cup | 225 | | 102 | 23 | 13 |
| **Cereals—Hot (Cooked without Adding Salt)** | | | | | | |
| Cream of Wheat, instant—Nabisco | 1 pkg | 9 | 35 | 100 | 21 | 0 |
| Cream of Wheat, quick—Nabisco | 1 pkg | 90 | 40 | 100 | 21 | 0 |
| Cream of Wheat, regular—Nabisco | 1 pkg | 7 | 35 | 100 | 21 | 0 |
| Farina, cooked | 1 cup | 2 | | 140 | 30 | 0 |
| Maltex, cooked | 1 cup | 1 | | 147 | 32 | 0.5 |
| Malt-O-Meal, cooked | 1 cup | 1 | 21 | 135 | 29 | 0.3 |
| Mix 'n Eat, cream of wheat—Nabisco | 1 pkg | 235 | 40 | 100 | 21 | 0 |
| Mix 'n Eat, baked apple with cinnamon flavor | 1 pkg | 255 | 50 | 130 | 29 | 0 |
| Mix 'n Eat banana flavor—Nabisco | 1 pkg | 255 | 50 | 130 | 29 | 0 |
| Mix 'n Eat, apple flavor and brown sugar | 1 pkg | 310 | 60 | 130 | 29 | 0 |
| oatmeal, cooked | 1 cup | 0.8 | 130 | 148 | 26 | 3 |
| pablum, barley, cooked | 1 cup | 491 | | 133 | 29 | 0.4 |
| pablum, rice, cooked | 1 cup | 397 | | 133 | 31 | 0.4 |
| Pep—Kellogg's, cooked | 1 cup | 226 | | 106 | 24 | 0.4 |

| | | | | | | |
|---|---|---|---|---|---|---|
| Pettijohn's wheat | 1 cup | 9 | | 150 | 32 | 0.9 |
| Ralston | 1 cup | 0.5 | | 141 | 30 | 0.9 |
| Wheatena | 1 cup | 0.9 | | 152 | 33 | 0.9 |
| **Cereals—Especially Prepared for Low-Sodium Diets** | | | | | | |
| Cornflakes—Cellu | 1 oz | <10 | | 110 | 25 | 0 |
| Cornflakes—Van Brode | 1 oz | 10 | | 110 | 25 | 0 |
| Corn, puffed—Nu-Vita | 1 oz | 2 | | | | |
| Millet, puffed—Nu-Vita | 1 oz | 2 | | | | |
| Pernola, unsalted—Flavor Tree Foods Inc. | 1 oz | 1 | | 126 | 15 | 5 |
| Rice Krispies—Van Brode | 1 oz | 10 | | 110 | 26 | 0 |
| Rice, puffed—Nu-Vita | 1 oz | 2 | | | | |
| Wheat, puffed—Nu-Vita | 1 oz | 2 | | | | |
| **Corn Products—Flour** | | | | | | |
| barley flour | 1 cup | 3 | 179 | 401 | 86 | 2 |
| buckwheat flour—dark | 1 cup | 1 | 656 | 333 | 72 | 3 |
| corn flour | 1 cup | 1 | | 405 | 85 | 3 |
| corn meal | 1 cup | 1628 | 276 | 409 | 85 | 4 |
| corn starch | ¼ cup | tr | tr | 181 | 44 | tr |
| rye flour | 1 cup | 1 | 125 | 286 | 62 | 1 |
| soy flour | 1 cup | 1 | 1195 | 303 | 22 | 15 |

| CATEGORY & FOOD | PORTION | SODIUM (mg) | POTAS-SIUM (mg) | CALO-RIES | CARBO-HYDRATES (g) | FAT (g) |
|---|---|---|---|---|---|---|
| wheat flour | 1 cup | 2 | 105 | 400 | 84 | 1 |
| whole wheat flour | 1 cup | 4 | 444 | 400 | 85 | 2 |
| **Cereal Products—Pasta and Grain** | | | | | | |
| corn grits, cooked without salt | 1 cup | tr | 27 | 123 | 27 | 0.2 |
| macaroni, cooked without salt | 1 cup | 1 | 110 | 207 | 42 | 0.7 |
| noodles, egg, cooked without salt | 1 cup | 3 | 70 | 200 | 37 | 2 |
| rice, brown, cooked without salt | 1 cup | 3 | 105 | 178 | 38 | 0.9 |
| rice, instant, cooked without salt | 1 cup | tr | tr | 161 | 36 | tr |
| rice, long-grain, cooked without salt | 1 cup | 3 | 65 | 159 | 35 | 0.2 |
| rice, white, milled, cooked without salt | 1 cup | 3 | 42 | 164 | 36 | 0.2 |
| spaghetti, cooked without salt | 1 cup | 1 | 115 | 216 | 44 | 0.7 |
| wheat germ | 1 tbsp | tr | 83 | 36 | 5 | 1 |
| wild rice | ¼ cup | 2 | 62 | 99 | 21 | 0.2 |
| **Cereal Products—Pasta and Grain Dishes** | | | | | | |
| beef ravioli | 7½ oz | 958 | | 240 | 34 | 7 |
| lasagna | 8 oz | 545 | | 208 | 12 | 13 |
| macaroni and cheese, baked | 7 oz | 608 | 116 | 200 | 21 | 8 |

| | | | | | | |
|---|---|---|---|---|---|---|
| spaghetti in tomato sauce with cheese | 7 oz | 764 | 326 | 208 | 29 | 7 |
| spaghetti with meatballs in tomato sauce | 7 oz | 814 | 536 | 268 | 29 | 7 |
| Spanish rice | 1 cup | 475 | 347 | 130 | 25 | 3 |
| **Cereal Products—Pasta and Grain Dishes Especially Prepared for Low-Sodium Diets** | | | | | | |
| Beef ravioli—Featherweight | 8 oz | 100 | | 230 | 35 | 6 |
| Spaghetti with meatballs—Featherweight | 8 oz | 55 | | 200 | 24 | 8 |
| Spanish rice—Featherweight | 7¼ oz | 31 | | 140 | 28 | 1 |
| **Dairy Products** | | | | | | |
| butter, salted | 1 tbsp | 138 | 3 | 100 | tr | 11 |
| butter, unsalted | 1 tbsp | 1 | 3 | 105 | tr | 11 |
| cheese, American | 1 oz | 318 | 22 | 107 | 0.5 | 8 |
| cheese, cheddar | 1 oz | 197 | 23 | 112 | 0.6 | 9 |
| cheese, cream | 1 oz | 70 | 21 | 105 | 0.6 | 11 |
| cheese, creamed cottage | ½ cup | 258 | 96 | 120 | 3 | 5 |
| cheese, Parmesan | 1 oz | 205 | 42 | 110 | 0.8 | 7 |
| cheese, processed, American | 1 oz | 318 | 22 | 107 | 0.5 | 8 |
| cheese, processed, Swiss | 1 oz | 327 | 28 | 100 | 0.4 | 8 |
| cheese, spread, American | 4 tsp | 285 | | 60 | 60 | 14 |
| cheese, spread, w bacon artif. flavor | 4 tsp | 240 | | 60 | 60 | 14 |
| cheese, spread, cheddar | 4 tsp | 235 | | 60 | 60 | 14 |
| cheese, spread, chive 'n green onion flavor | 4 tsp | 255 | | 55 | 60 | 14 |

| CATEGORY & FOOD | PORTION | SODIUM (mg) | POTASSIUM (mg) | CALORIES | CARBOHYDRATES (g) | FAT (g) |
|---|---|---|---|---|---|---|
| cheese, spread w French onion flavor | 4 tsp | 250 | | 60 | 60 | 14 |
| cheese, spread, hickory smoke flavor | 4 tsp | 250 | | 60 | 60 | 14 |
| cheese, spread, w pimiento | 4 tsp | 250 | | 60 | 60 | 14 |
| cheese, spread, sharp cheddar | 4 tsp | 295 | | 60 | 60 | 14 |
| cheese, Swiss | 1 oz | 199 | 29 | 106 | 0.5 | 8 |
| cream, heavy | 1 tbsp | 5 | 13 | 52 | 0.5 | 6 |
| cream, powdered | 1 tsp | 17 | | 15 | 2 | 0.8 |
| cream, sour | 1 oz | 13 | | 57 | 1 | 5 |
| cream, table | 1 tbsp | 6 | 18 | 32 | 0.6 | 3 |
| Ice cream, diet-Weight Watchers | ½ pint | 109 | | 163 | 31 | 2 |
| Ice cream, regular, aver. | ½ pint | 86 | 245 | 261 | 28 | 14 |
| margarine | 1 tbsp | 138 | 3 | 101 | 0 | 11 |
| margarine, salt-free | 1 tbsp | 1 | | 100 | 0 | 11 |
| milk, buttermilk | 8 oz | 215 | 388 | 81 | 10 | 0.2 |
| milk, condensed | 1 tbsp | 22 | 63 | 64 | 11 | 2 |
| milk, dried | 1 tbsp | 28 | 93 | 35 | 3 | 2 |
| milk, evaporated | 1 tbsp | 19 | 49 | 22 | 2 | 1 |
| milk, goat | 1 cup | 83 | 439 | 163 | 11 | 10 |
| milk, human | 4 oz | 20 | 60 | 92 | 11 | 5 |
| milk, skim | 1 tbsp | 8 | 22 | 5 | 0.8 | tr |
| milk, skim | 8 oz | 128 | 356 | 88 | 13 | 0.2 |

| | | | | | | |
|---|---|---|---|---|---|---|
| milk, whole | 1 tbsp | 8 | 22 | 10 | 0.7 | 0.5 |
| milk, whole | 8 oz | 127 | 356 | 161 | 12 | 9 |
| yogurt, regular | 1 cup | 124 | 349 | 122 | 13 | 4 |
| yogurt, skim | 1 cup | 115 | 322 | 151 | 12 | 8 |
| **Dairy Products—Especially Prepared for Low-Sodium Diets** | | | | | | |
| Cheese, Cheddar—Cellu | 1 oz | 5 | | 110 | 0 | 9 |
| Cheese, Cheddar, salt-free—Redwood Natural | 1 oz | 4 | | | | |
| Cheese, Colby—Cellu | 1 oz | 5 | | 110 | 0 | 9 |
| Cheese, Colby low-sodium—Pauly | 1 oz | 6 | | | | |
| Cheese, Cottage—Daitch Shopwell | 1 oz | 3 | | | | |
| Cheese, Dutch Gouda | 1 oz | 12 | | | | |
| Cheese, Jack, salt-free—Redwood Natural | 1 oz | 5 | | | | |
| Cheese, Muenster, unsalted—Ralph's | 1 oz | 6 | | | | |
| Milk, nonfat, dry, low-sodium—Featherweight | 8 oz mixed | 6 | | 70 | 10 | 0 |
| **Desserts** | | | | | | |
| Gelatin, dry, plain | 1 tbsp | 11 | 0.2 | 34 | 0 | 0 |
| Gelatin, cherry—Jell-o | ½ cup | 55 | 1 | 80 | 18 | 0 |
| Gelatin, lime—Jell-o | ½ cup | 57 | 2 | 80 | 18 | 0 |
| Gelatin, orange—Jell-o | ½ cup | 51 | 2 | 80 | 19 | 0 |

| CATEGORY & FOOD | PORTION | SODIUM (mg) | POTASSIUM (mg) | CALORIES | CARBOHYDRATES (g) | FAT (g) |
|---|---|---|---|---|---|---|
| Gelatin, raspberry—Jell-o | ½ cup | 49 | 2 | 80 | 18 | 0 |
| Gelatin, strawberry—Jell-o | ½ cup | 51 | 1 | 80 | 18 | 0 |
| Gelatin, wild cherry—Jell-o | ½ cup | 73 | 1 | 80 | 18 | 0 |
| Gelatin, wild strawberry—Jell-o | ½ cup | 100 | 1 | 80 | 18 | 0 |
| ice cream, chocolate | ½ pint | 75 | | 300 | 33 | 16 |
| ice cream, chocolate covered | 1 bar | 28 | | 162 | 15 | 11 |
| ice cream, strawberry | ½ pint | 60 | | 254 | 32 | 12 |
| ice cream, vanilla | ½ pint | 82 | | 290 | 30 | 16 |
| ice cream cone | 1 cone | 28 | 29 | 45 | 9 | 0.3 |
| Ice Cream Cone, Comet—Nabisco | 1 cone | 5 | 5 | 18 | 4 | 0 |
| Ice Cream Comet cups—Nabisco | 1 cup | 5 | 5 | 18 | 4 | 0 |
| ice milk, chocolate | ½ pint | 92 | 263 | 206 | 30 | 7 |
| ice milk, chocolate covered | 1 bar | 38 | | 144 | 16 | 8 |
| ice milk, strawberry | ½ pint | 96 | | 200 | 33 | 5 |
| ice milk, vanilla | ½ pint | 113 | | 204 | 31 | 11 |
| ices, orange | ½ pint | tr | 6 | 144 | 60 | tr |
| Pudding, Butterscotch—Cool 'n Creamy | ½ cup | 185 | 188 | 170 | 30 | 5 |
| Pudding, Dark chocolate—Cool 'n Creamy | ½ cup | 222 | 258 | 190 | 31 | 5 |
| Pudding, Light chocolate—Cool 'n Creamy | ½ cup | 204 | 208 | 180 | 30 | 5 |
| Pudding, Vanilla—Cool 'n Creamy | ½ cup | 186 | 187 | 170 | 28 | 5 |
| Pudding, Low-Calorie, Butterscotch—D-Zerta | ½ cup | 164 | 215 | 70 | 13 | 0 |

| | | | | | | |
|---|---|---|---|---|---|---|
| Pudding, Low-Calorie, Chocolate—D-Zerta | ½ cup | 100 | 227 | 70 | 12 | 0 |
| Pudding, Low-Calorie, Vanilla—D-Zerta | ½ cup | 139 | 222 | 70 | 13 | 0 |
| rice pudding with raisins | ¾ cup | 103 | 257 | 212 | 39 | 5 |
| sherbet, orange | 1 serving | 10 | 22 | 134 | 31 | 1 |
| tapioca, apple | ½ cup | 62 | 32 | 143 | 36 | 0.1 |
| tapioca, cream | ½ cup | 203 | 176 | 174 | 22 | 0.7 |
| **Desserts—Especially Prepared for Low-Sodium Diets** | | | | | | |
| Gelatin, various fruit flav.—D-Zerta | ½ cup | 4 | 50 | 8 | 0 | 0 |
| Gelatin, fruit flavored—Featherweight | ½ cup | 5 | | 10 | 0 | 0 |
| Gelatin, fruit flavored—Van Winkle | ½ cup | 5 | | 8 | | 0 |
| Pudding, butterscotch—Featherweight | ½ cup | 20 | | 12 | 3 | 0 |
| Pudding, chocolate—Featherweight | ½ cup | 25 | | 25 | 4 | 1 |
| Pudding, vanilla—Featherweight | ½ cup | 15 | | 12 | 3 | 0 |
| **Eggs** | | | | | | |
| Egg Beaters | ¼ cup | 109 | 128 | 100 | | <1 |
| egg white | 1 medium | 47 | 43 | 16 | 0.3 | tr |
| egg, whole | 1 medium | 59 | 62 | 78 | 0.4 | 6 |
| egg yolk | 1 medium | 12 | 19 | 59 | 0.1 | 5 |
| **Fats and Oils** | | | | | | |
| butter, salted | 1 tbsp | 138 | 3 | 100 | 0.1 | 11 |

| CATEGORY & FOOD | PORTION | SODIUM (mg) | POTASSIUM (mg) | CALORIES | CARBOHYDRATES (g) | FAT (g) |
|---|---|---|---|---|---|---|
| butter, unsalted | 1 tbsp | 1 | 3 | 100 | 0.1 | 11 |
| coconut cream | 1 tbsp | 1 | 45 | 47 | 1 | 5 |
| corn oil | 1 tbsp | 0 | 0 | 126 | 0 | 14 |
| cottonseed oil | 1 tbsp | 0 | 0 | 126 | 0 | 14 |
| lard | 1 tbsp | 0 | 0 | 126 | 0 | 14 |
| margarine—diet | 1 tbsp | 76 | | 50 | 0 | 6 |
| margarine—salted | 1 tbsp | 138 | 3 | 100 | 0.1 | 11 |
| margarine—unsalted | 1 tbsp | 1 | | 100 | 0 | 11 |
| olive oil | 1 tbsp | 0 | 0 | 124 | 0 | 14 |
| peanut oil | 1 tbsp | 0 | 0 | 124 | 0 | 14 |
| safflower oil | 1 tbsp | 0 | 0 | 124 | 0 | 14 |
| salt pork | ¼ lb slab | 1370 | 47 | 885 | 0 | 96 |
| soybean oil | 1 tbsp | 0 | 0 | 124 | 0 | 14 |
| **Fish and Seafood—Uncooked** | | | | | | |
| bass, sea | 4 oz | 78 | 287 | 106 | 0 | 1 |
| bluefish | 4 oz | 85 | | 134 | 0 | 4 |
| carp | 4 oz | 57 | 327 | 131 | 0 | 5 |
| catfish | 4 oz | 69 | 377 | 118 | 0 | 4 |
| clams, hard | 10 small | 205 | 311 | 80 | 6 | 0.9 |

| | | | | | | |
|---|---|---|---|---|---|---|
| clams, soft | 9 small | 36 | 235 | 82 | 1 | 2 |
| cod | 4 oz | 80 | 437 | 89 | 0 | 0.3 |
| croaker | 4 oz | 99 | 267 | 110 | 0 | 3 |
| drum, fresh water | 4 oz | 80 | 329 | 138 | 0 | 6 |
| drum, red | 4 oz | 63 | 312 | 91 | 0 | 0.5 |
| flatfish | 4 oz | 89 | 391 | 90 | 0 | 0.9 |
| flounder | 4 oz | 89 | 391 | 90 | 0 | 0.9 |
| haddock | 4 oz | 70 | 347 | 90 | 0 | 0.1 |
| hake | 4 oz | 85 | 415 | 85 | 0 | 0.5 |
| halibut | 4 oz | 62 | 513 | 114 | 0 | 1 |
| herring, Pacific | 4 oz | 85 | 480 | 112 | 0 | 3 |
| kingfish | 4 oz | 95 | 286 | 120 | 0 | 3 |
| lake herring | 4 oz | 54 | 365 | 110 | 0 | 3 |
| ling cod | 4 oz | 67 | 495 | 96 | 0 | 0.9 |
| lobster | 4 oz | 230 | | 104 | 2.17 | .57 |
| mullet, striped | 4 oz | 93 | 334 | 167 | 0 | 8 |
| mussels, meat | 4 oz | 330 | 360 | 109 | 4 | 3 |
| ocean perch | 4 oz | 72 | 446 | 109 | 0 | 2 |
| oysters | 5-8 medium | 73 | 121 | 66 | 3 | 2 |
| perch, yellow | 4 oz | 78 | 263 | 104 | 0 | 1 |
| pike, walleye | 4 oz | 58 | 365 | 106 | 0 | 1 |
| pollock | 4 oz | 55 | 400 | 109 | 0 | 1 |
| pompano | 4 oz | 54 | 218 | 190 | 0 | 11 |
| porgy | 4 oz | 72 | 328 | 128 | 0 | 4 |

| CATEGORY & FOOD | PORTION | SODIUM (mg) | POTAS-SIUM (mg) | CALO-RIES | CARBO-HYDRATES (g) | FAT (g) |
|---|---|---|---|---|---|---|
| red and gray snapper | 4 oz | 77 | 369 | 108 | 0 | 1 |
| rockfish | 4 oz | 69 | 443 | 111 | 0 | 2 |
| sablefish | 4 oz | 64 | 409 | 217 | 0 | 17 |
| salmon, chinook | 4 oz | 51 | 456 | 254 | 0 | 18 |
| salmon, pink | 4 oz | 73 | 350 | 136 | 0 | 4 |
| salmon, sockeye | 4 oz | 55 | 447 | | | |
| scallops—frozen in brine | 4 oz | 291 | 453 | 93 | 4 | 0.2 |
| shad | 4 oz | 62 | 377 | 194 | 0 | 11 |
| sheepshead | 4 oz | 115 | 267 | 129 | 0 | 3 |
| shrimp | 4 oz | 160 | 251 | 104 | 2 | 0.9 |
| sole | 4 oz | 89 | 391 | 90 | 0 | 0.9 |
| Spanish mackerel | 4 oz | 78 | 302 | 202 | 0 | 12 |
| spot | 4 oz | 70 | | 250 | 0 | 18 |
| sucker | 4 oz | 64 | 384 | 119 | 0 | 2 |
| tuna, yellow fin | 4 oz | 42 | | 152 | 0 | 3 |
| weakfish | 4 oz | 86 | 362 | 138 | 0 | 6 |
| whitefish, lake | 4 oz | 59 | 342 | 177 | 0 | 9 |
| **Fish and Seafood—Canned** | | | | | | |
| caviar | 1 rnd. tsp | 22 | 18 | 32 | 1 | 2 |

| | | | | | | |
|---|---|---|---|---|---|---|
| crabmeat | ½ cup | 850 | 94 | 86 | 0.9 | 2 |
| lobster meat | 4 oz | 240 | 206 | 109 | 0.3 | 2 |
| salmon, pink | ½ cup | 484 | 451 | 176 | 0 | 7 |
| salmon, sockeye | ½ cup | 653 | 430 | 214 | 0 | 12 |
| sardines, mustard or brine | 4 oz | 869 | 297 | 224 | 2 | 14 |
| sardines, tomato sauce | 4 oz | 457 | 366 | 225 | 2 | 14 |
| tuna, oil | ½ cup | 533 | 200 | 192 | 0 | 14 |
| tuna, water | ½ cup | 41 | 279 | 127 | 0 | 0.8 |
| **Fish and Seafood—Canned Especially Prepared for Low-Sodium Diets** | | | | | | |
| Gefilte fish, unsalted—Mother's | 1 ball | 3 | | | | |
| Mackerel, fillets—Roland | 3 oz | 49 | | | | |
| Salmon—Arcadia | ½ cup | 53 | | 181 | | |
| Salmon—Balanced | ½ cup | 50 | | 79 | | 5 |
| Salmon—Featherweight | ½ can | 65 | | | | |
| Salmon—S & W Nutradiet | ½ cup | 47 | | | | |
| Sardines—Arcadia | 3 oz | 64 | | | | |
| Sardines—Beatriz | 3 oz | 49 | | | | |
| Sardines—Cellu | 3 oz | 103 | | | | |
| Sardines—King Roland | 3 oz | 94 | | | | |
| Sardines—Lilly Brand | 3 oz | 35 | | | | |
| Sardines in oil—Cellu | 3 oz | 103 | | | | |

| CATEGORY & FOOD | PORTION | SODIUM (mg) | POTASSIUM (mg) | CALORIES | CARBOHYDRATES (g) | FAT (g) |
|---|---|---|---|---|---|---|
| Sardines in tomato sauce—Cellu | 3 oz | 103 | | | | |
| Tuna fish—Arcadia | ½ cup | 34 | | 91 | | 1 |
| Tuna fish—Balanced | 4 oz | 40 | | 120 | 0.2 | 0.6 |
| Tuna fish—Chicken of the Sea | ½ cup | 34 | | 91 | | 1 |
| Tuna fish—Featherweight | ½ can | 37 | | 120 | 0 | 2 |
| **Fruits—Uncooked (Raw, Frozen and Dried)** | | | | | | |
| apples | 1 medium | 1 | 165 | 87 | 22 | 0.9 |
| apples, frozen, sugar added | ½ cup | 14 | 68 | 93 | 24 | 0.1 |
| apricots | 2-3 medium | 1 | 281 | 51 | 13 | 0.2 |
| apricots, dried | 8 halves, lg | 13 | 490 | 130 | 33 | 0.3 |
| avocado, peeled, pitted | ½ cup | 4 | 604 | 167 | 6 | 16 |
| banana | 1 medium | 2 | 550 | 127 | 33 | 0.3 |
| blackberries | ½ cup | 0.5 | 122 | 42 | 9 | 0.7 |
| blackberries, frozen, no sugar | ½ cup | 0.5 | 115 | 36 | 9 | 0.3 |
| blueberries | ½ cup | 0.5 | 57 | 44 | 11 | 0.4 |
| blueberries, frozen, no sugar | ½ cup | 0.5 | 65 | 44 | 11 | 0.4 |
| blueberries, frozen, sugar added | ½ cup | 0.5 | 50 | 77 | 20 | 0.5 |
| boysenberries, frozen, no sugar | ½ cup | 0.1 | 96 | 30 | 7 | 0.2 |
| boysenberries, frozen, sugar added | ½ cup | 0.5 | 79 | 72 | 18 | 0.2 |

| | | | | | | |
|---|---|---|---|---|---|---|
| cantaloupe | ¼ melon | 12 | 251 | 30 | 8 | 0.1 |
| cherries, red sour | ½ cup | 2 | 191 | 58 | 14 | 0.3 |
| cherries, red sour, frozen, no sugar | ½ cup | 2 | 188 | 55 | 13 | 0.4 |
| cherries, red sour, frozen, sugar added | ½ cup | 2 | 130 | 112 | 28 | 0.4 |
| cherries, sweet | 10 medium | 1 | 96 | 35 | 9 | 0.2 |
| cranberries | ½ cup | 1 | 41 | 23 | 5 | 0.4 |
| currants, black | ½ cup | 2 | 248 | 36 | 9 | 0.1 |
| currants, white and red | ½ cup | 1 | 171 | 33 | 8 | 0.1 |
| dates, domestic, pitted | 10 | 1 | 648 | 274 | 73 | 0.5 |
| dates, dried, pitted, cut | ½ cup | 1 | 575 | 244 | 65 | 0.5 |
| figs, dried | 3 small | 15 | 288 | 123 | 31 | 0.6 |
| figs, fresh | 3 small | 2 | 194 | 80 | 20 | 0.3 |
| gooseberries | ½ cup | 0.8 | 116 | 29 | 7 | 0.2 |
| granadilla, purple | 3½ oz | 28 | 348 | 90 | 21 | 0.7 |
| grapefruit, pink | ½ medium | 1 | 135 | 40 | 10 | 0.1 |
| grapefruit, white | ½ medium | 1 | 135 | 41 | 11 | 0.1 |
| grapes, adherent | ½ cup | 3 | 139 | 54 | 14 | 0.3 |
| grapes, American | 22 medium | 3 | 158 | 69 | 16 | 1 |
| grapes, European | 24 medium | 3 | 173 | 67 | 17 | 0.3 |
| grapes, slipskin | ½ cup | 3 | 121 | 53 | 12 | 0.8 |
| guava, common | 1 medium | 4 | 289 | 62 | 15 | 0.6 |
| honeydew melon | ¼ small | 12 | 251 | 33 | 8 | 0.3 |
| kumquats | 5 medium | 7 | 236 | 65 | 17 | 0.7 |

| CATEGORY & FOOD | PORTION | SODIUM (mg) | POTASSIUM (mg) | CALORIES | CARBOHYDRATES (g) | FAT (g) |
|---|---|---|---|---|---|---|
| lemons, peeled | 1 medium | 2 | 138 | 27 | 8 | 0.3 |
| limes | 1 medium | 2 | 102 | 28 | 10 | 0.2 |
| litchis | 3½ oz | 3 | 170 | 64 | 16 | 0.3 |
| loganberries | ½ cup | 0.8 | 128 | 47 | 6 | 0.5 |
| mangoes | ½ medium | 7 | 189 | 66 | 17 | 0.4 |
| mulberries | ½ cup | 0.8 | 150 | 47 | 11 | 0.5 |
| nectarines | 1 medium | 3 | 147 | 32 | 9 | tr |
| olives, Greek | 1 medium | 219 | | 22 | 0.6 | 3 |
| olives, pickled | 1 medium | 156 | 4 | 8 | 0.1 | 0.8 |
| oranges | 1 medium | 2 | 300 | 73 | 18 | 0.3 |
| papayas | ½ medium | 5 | 351 | 54 | 15 | 0.2 |
| peaches | 1 meduim | 1 | 202 | 38 | 10 | 0.1 |
| peaches, dried, sugar added | ½ cup | 13 | 760 | 210 | 63 | 0.6 |
| peaches, sliced, frozen, sugar added | ½ cup | 3 | 155 | 110 | 28 | 0.1 |
| pears | 1 medium | 4 | 260 | 122 | 31 | 0.8 |
| persimmons—Japanese | 1 medium | 6 | 174 | 77 | 20 | 0.4 |
| persimmons—native | 1 medium | 1 | 310 | 127 | 34 | 0.4 |
| pineapple | 1 slice | 1 | 123 | 44 | 12 | 0.2 |
| pineapple, frozen, chunks | ½ cup | 3 | 133 | 113 | 30 | 0.1 |
| plantain | 1 small | 5 | 385 | 119 | 31 | 0.4 |

| | | | | | | |
|---|---|---|---|---|---|---|
| plums, damson | 1 medium | 1 | 150 | 33 | 9 | tr |
| pomegranate | 1 medium | 3 | 259 | 63 | 16 | 0.3 |
| prunes, dehydrated | 1 large | 1 | 118 | 43 | 11 | 0.1 |
| prunes, dried | 1 large | 0.8 | 69 | 26 | 7 | 0.1 |
| quinces | 3½ oz | 4 | 197 | 57 | 15 | 0.1 |
| raisins, seeded, dried | ½ cup | 19 | 542 | 205 | 55 | 0.2 |
| raisins, seedless, dried | ½ cup | 22 | 610 | 231 | 62 | 0.2 |
| raspberries, black | ½ cup | 0.8 | 150 | 52 | 12 | 1 |
| raspberries, red | ½ cup | 0.7 | 112 | 38 | 91 | 0.3 |
| raspberries, red, frozen, sugar added | ½ cup | 1 | 123 | 121 | 30 | 0.2 |
| rhubarb | ½ cup | 1 | 126 | 8 | 2 | 0.1 |
| rhubarb, frozen, sugar added | ½ cup | 4 | 235 | 157 | 48 | 0.3 |
| sapodilla | ½ cup | 12 | 193 | 89 | 22 | 1 |
| strawberries, stems removed, whole | ½ cup | 1 | 123 | 28 | 6 | 0.4 |
| strawberries, whole, frozen, sugar added | ½ cup | 1 | 127 | 112 | 29 | 0.2 |
| tamarind | 3½ oz | 51 | 781 | 239 | 63 | 0.6 |
| tangerine | 1 large | 2 | 126 | 46 | 12 | 0.2 |
| tomato | 1 small | 3 | 244 | 22 | 5 | 0.2 |
| watermelon | 1 slice | 6 | 600 | 156 | 38 | 1 |
| watermelon balls | ½ cup | 1 | 100 | 26 | 6 | 0.2 |

| | | | | | | |
|---|---|---|---|---|---|---|
| **Fruits—Canned** | | | | | | |
| applecubes, artificially sweetened | ½ cup | 3 | | 25 | 6 | 0.1 |

| CATEGORY & FOOD | PORTION | SODIUM (mg) | POTASSIUM (mg) | CALORIES | CARBOHYDRATES (g) | FAT (g) |
|---|---|---|---|---|---|---|
| applesauce, sugar added | ½ cup | 2 | 65 | 91 | 24 | 0.1 |
| applesauce, no sugar | ½ cup | 2 | 78 | 41 | 11 | 0.2 |
| applesauce, artificially sweetened | ½ cup | 2 | 78 | 41 | 11 | 0.2 |
| apricots, water packed, no sugar | 3 med halves | 1 | 246 | 38 | 10 | 0.1 |
| apricots, water packed, artificially swt. | 3 med halves | 1 | 246 | 38 | 10 | 0.1 |
| apricots, juice packed, sugar added | 3 med halves | 1 | 362 | 54 | 14 | 0.2 |
| apricots, heavy syrup, sugar added | 3 med halves | 1 | 234 | 86 | 22 | 0.1 |
| blackberries, water packed, no sugar | ½ cup | 1 | 144 | 50 | 10 | 0.8 |
| blackberries, water packed, artificially swt. | ½ cup | 1 | 144 | 50 | 10 | 0.8 |
| blackberries, juice packed | ½ cup | 1 | 213 | 68 | 15 | 1 |
| blackberries, heavy syrup, sugar added | ½ cup | 1 | 136 | 114 | 18 | 0.8 |
| blueberries, water packed, artificially swt. | ½ cup | 1 | 73 | 47 | 12 | 0.2 |
| blueberries, heavy syrup, sugar added | ½ cup | 1 | 66 | 121 | 31 | 0.2 |
| cherries, sour, water packed, no sugar | ½ cup | 2 | 130 | 43 | 11 | 0.2 |
| cherries, sour, heavy syrup, sugar added | ½ cup | 1 | 124 | 89 | 23 | 0.2 |
| cherries, sweet, water packed, no sugar | ½ cup | 2 | 130 | 43 | 11 | 0.2 |
| cherries, sweet, heavy syrup, sugar added | ½ cup | 1 | 124 | 89 | 23 | 0.2 |
| cranberry sauce | ½ cup | 1 | 41 | 199 | 51 | 0.3 |
| figs, water packed, no sugar | 3 med | 2 | 155 | 48 | 12 | 0.2 |
| figs, heavy syrup, sugar added | 3 med | 2 | 149 | 84 | 22 | 0.2 |

| | | | | | | |
|---|---|---|---|---|---|---|
| fruit cocktail, water packed, no sugar | ½ cup | 5 | 168 | 37 | 10 | 0.1 |
| fruit cocktail, heavy syrup, sugar added | ½ cup | 5 | 161 | 76 | 20 | 0.1 |
| gooseberries, water packed, no sugar | ½ cup | 1 | 105 | 26 | 7 | 0.9 |
| gooseberries, heavy syrup, sugar added | ½ cup | 1 | 98 | 90 | 23 | 0.1 |
| grapefruit, water packed, no sugar | ½ cup | 4 | 144 | 30 | 8 | 0.1 |
| grapefruit, syrup, sugar added | ½ cup | 1 | 135 | 70 | 18 | 0.1 |
| loganberries, water packed, no sugar | ½ cup | 1 | 115 | 40 | 9 | 0.4 |
| loganberries, heavy syrup, sugar added | ½ cup | 1 | 109 | 89 | 22 | 0.4 |
| peaches, water packed, no sugar | ½ cup | 2 | 137 | 31 | 8 | 0.1 |
| peaches, juice packed | 2 med halves | 2 | 205 | 45 | 12 | 0.1 |
| peaches, heavy syrup, sugar added | 2 med halves | 2 | 130 | 78 | 20 | 0.1 |
| pears, water packed, no sugar | ½ cup | 1 | 110 | 40 | 10 | 0.3 |
| pears, heavy syrup, sugar added | 2 halves | 1 | 84 | 76 | 20 | 0.2 |
| pineapple, water packed, no sugar | 1 lg sl & ju | 1 | 99 | 39 | 10 | 0.1 |
| pineapple, juice packed | 1 lg sl & ju | 1 | 147 | 58 | 15 | 0.1 |
| pineapple, syrup, sugar added | 1 lg sl & ju | 1 | 96 | 74 | 19 | 0.1 |
| plums, green gage, water packed, no sugar | 4 oz | 1 | 94 | 38 | 10 | 0.1 |
| plums, purple, water packed, no sugar | 4 oz | 2 | 167 | 52 | 14 | 0.2 |
| plums, purple, heavy syrup, sugar added | ½ cup | 1 | 166 | 97 | 25 | 0.1 |
| pumpkin | ½ cup | 3 | 300 | 41 | 10 | 0.4 |
| raspberries, black, water packed, no sugar | ½ cup | 1 | 135 | 51 | 11 | 1 |
| raspberries, red, water packed, no sugar | ½ cup | 1 | 114 | 35 | 9 | 0.1 |
| strawberries, water packed | ½ cup | 1 | 148 | 29 | 7 | 0.1 |

| CATEGORY & FOOD | PORTION | SODIUM (mg) | POTASSIUM (mg) | CALORIES | CARBOHYDRATES (g) | FAT (g) |
|---|---|---|---|---|---|---|
| **Fruits—Canned—Especially Prepared for Low-Sodium Diets** | | | | | | |
| Applesauce—Arcadia | ½ cup | 3 | | 60 | 14 | 0 |
| Applesauce—Balanced | 4 oz | 2 | | 48 | 10 | 0.4 |
| Applesauce—Featherweight | ½ cup | 10 | | 50 | 13 | 0 |
| Applesauce—Tillie Lewis | ½ cup | <10 | | 60 | 15 | 0 |
| Apricots—Arcadia | ½ cup | 5 | | 35 | 9 | 0 |
| Apricots—Balanced | ½ cup | 3 | | 44 | 10 | 0.1 |
| Apricots—Cellu | ½ cup | 3 | | 35 | 9 | 0 |
| Apricots—Featherweight | ½ cup | 3 | | 50 | 13 | 0 |
| Apricots—Tillie Lewis | ½ cup | 10 | | 60 | 15 | 0 |
| Blackberries—Balanced | 4 oz | 1 | | 48 | 10 | 0.4 |
| Blueberries—Balanced | 4 oz | 0.8 | | 48 | 10 | 0.4 |
| Blueberries—Featherweight | ½ cup | 2 | | 41 | 11 | 0 |
| Cherries, dark sweet—Balanced | 4 oz | 1 | | 54 | 13 | 0.1 |
| Cherries, dark sweet—Cellu | ½ cup | 3 | | 57 | 13 | 0 |
| Cherries, light sweet—Tillie Lewis | ½ cup | <10 | | 60 | 14 | 0 |
| Cherries, light sweet—Cellu | ½ cup | 1 | | 48 | 11 | 0 |
| Cherries, Royal Ann—Balanced | 4 oz | 1 | | 48 | 12 | 0.1 |
| Fruit cocktail—Arcadia | ½ cup | 6 | | 40 | 11 | 0 |
| Fruit cocktail—Balanced | 4 oz | 1 | | 36 | 9 | 0.1 |

| | | | | | |
|---|---|---|---|---|---|
| Fruit cocktail—Cellu | ½ cup | 5 | 40 | 10 | 0 |
| Fruit cocktail—Featherweight | ½ cup | 5 | 50 | 14 | 0 |
| Fruit cocktail—Tillie Lewis | ½ cup | <10 | 50 | 13 | 0 |
| Fruits for salad—Cellu | ½ cup | 3 | 30 | 8 | 0 |
| Fruits for salad—Featherweight | ½ cup | 3 | 45 | 13 | 0 |
| Fruits for salad—Tillie Lewis | ½ cup | <10 | 60 | 15 | 0 |
| Grapefruit sections—Balanced | 4 oz | 1 | 40 | 8 | 0.1 |
| Grapefruit segments—Featherweight | ½ cup | 5 | 40 | 9 | 0 |
| Grapefruit—Tillie Lewis | ½ cup | <10 | 45 | 11 | 0 |
| Grapes, light, seedless—Cellu | ½ cup | 5 | 50 | 12 | 0 |
| Grapes, light, seedless—Featherweight | ½ cup | 5 | 50 | 12 | 0 |
| Kadota figs—Balanced | 4 oz | 3 | 45 | 10 | 0.3 |
| Kadota figs—Featherweight | ½ cup | 10 | 60 | 15 | 0 |
| Mandarin oranges—Featherweight | ½ cup | 5 | 30 | 6 | 0 |
| Mandarin oranges—Tillie Lewis | ½ cup | <10 | 45 | 11 | 0 |
| Peaches, Elberta—Tillie Lewis | ½ cup | 10 | 50 | 13 | 0 |
| Peaches, Freestone, halves—Featherweight | ½ cup | 8 | 50 | 14 | 0 |
| Peaches, Freestone, sliced—Featherweight | ½ cup | 8 | 50 | 14 | 0 |
| Peaches, yellow cling, halves—Arcadia | ½ cup | 5 | 30 | 8 | 0 |
| Peaches, yellow cling, sliced—Balanced | 4 oz | 3 | 24 | 6 | 0.1 |
| Peaches, yellow cling, halves—Cellu | ½ cup | 3 | 30 | 7 | 0 |
| Peaches, yellow cling, sliced—Cellu | ½ cup | 3 | 30 | 7 | 0 |
| Peaches, yellow cling, halves—Featherweight | ½ cup | 3 | 50 | 14 | 0 |

| CATEGORY & FOOD | PORTION | SODIUM (mg) | POTASSIUM (mg) | CALORIES | CARBOHYDRATES (g) | FAT (g) |
|---|---|---|---|---|---|---|
| Peaches, yellow cling, sliced—Featherweight | ½ cup | 3 | | 50 | 14 | 0 |
| Peaches, yellow cling—Tillie Lewis | ½ cup | 10 | | 45 | 13 | 0 |
| Peaches, sliced and pears—Featherweight | ½ cup | 3 | | 50 | 14 | 0 |
| Pears, Bartlett, halves—Cellu | ½ cup | 2 | | 37 | 9 | 0 |
| Pears, Bartlett, halves—Featherweight | ½ cup | 2 | | 57 | 14 | 0 |
| Pears, Bartlett—Tillie Lewis | ½ cup | <10 | | 50 | 13 | 0 |
| Pineapple chunks—Featherweight | ½ cup | 1 | | 70 | 18 | 0 |
| Pineapple, crushed—Featherweight | ½ cup | 1 | | 70 | 18 | 0 |
| Pineapple, sliced—Balanced | ½ cup | 2 | | 66 | 16 | 0 |
| Pineapple, sliced—Cellu | ½ cup | 1 | | 60 | 15 | 0 |
| Pineapple, sliced—Featherweight | ½ cup | 1 | | 70 | 18 | 0 |
| Pineapple—Tillie Lewis | ½ cup | <10 | | 70 | 18 | 0 |
| Pineapple tid bits—Featherweight | ½ cup | 1 | | 70 | 18 | 0 |
| Prunes, stewed—Featherweight | ½ cup | 8 | | 93 | 24 | 0 |
| Purple plums—Balanced | 4 oz | 1 | | 50 | 12 | 0.1 |
| Purple plums—Cellu | ½ cup | 2 | | 39 | 9 | 0 |
| Purple plums—Featherweight | ½ cup | 2 | | 67 | 18 | 0 |
| Purple plums—Tillie Lewis | ½ cup | <10 | | 70 | 18 | 0 |

| Fruit Drinks | | | | | | |
|---|---|---|---|---|---|---|
| Apple—Hi C | 6 oz | 12 | | 90 | 22 | 0 |
| Cherry—Hi C | 6 oz | 4 | | 90 | 23 | 0 |
| Citrus cooler—Hi C | 6 oz | 4 | | 90 | 23 | 0 |
| Grape—Hi C | 6 oz | 0 | | 115 | 28 | 0 |
| Grape flavored—Tang | 4 oz | 6 | 1 | 50 | 14 | 0 |
| Grapefruit flavored—Tang | 4 oz | 35 | 1 | 50 | 13 | 0 |
| Kool-Aid, all unsweetened flavors | 8 oz | 1 | 1 | 2 | 0 | 0 |
| Kool-Aid, fruit, sweetened | 8 oz | 1 | 1 | 90 | 23 | 0 |
| Kool-Aid, root beer flavored | 8 oz | 30 | 1 | 110 | 29 | 0 |
| Orange—Hi C | 6 oz | 58 | | 100 | 24 | 0 |
| Orange flavored—Tang | 4 oz | 7 | 31 | 50 | 13 | 0 |
| Orange Plus | 6 oz | 8 | 278 | 100 | 23 | 0 |
| Punch—Hi C | 6 oz | 3 | | 100 | 26 | 0 |
| Start | 4 oz | 47 | 47 | 50 | 13 | 0 |
| Strawberry cooler—Hi C | 6 oz | <1 | | 100 | 23 | 0 |
| Wild berry—Hi C | 6 oz | 5 | | 90 | 23 | 0 |

| Fruit Juices | | | | | | |
|---|---|---|---|---|---|---|
| Acerola juice | 4 oz | 4 | | 29 | 6 | 0.4 |
| apple cider, sweetened | 6 oz | 8 | 187 | 94 | 26 | 0 |
| apple juice, canned | 4 oz | 1 | 126 | 59 | 15 | tr |
| apricot, canned, unsweetened | 4 oz | 4 | | 61 | 15 | 0.1 |

| CATEGORY & FOOD | PORTION | SODIUM (mg) | POTASSIUM (mg) | CALORIES | CARBOHYDRATES (g) | FAT (g) |
|---|---|---|---|---|---|---|
| apricot nectar | 4 oz | 0.7 | 186 | 70 | 18 | 0.1 |
| blackberry, unsweetened | 4 oz | 1 | 212 | 46 | 10 | 0.8 |
| blueberry juice | 4 oz | 1 | 139 | 68 | 17 | 0 |
| cranberry cocktail | 4 oz | 1 | 125 | 81 | 21 | 0.1 |
| cranberry cocktail, low calorie | 4 oz | 4 | 125 | 25 | 6 | 0 |
| grapefruit, fresh | 4 oz | 1 | 203 | 49 | 12 | 0.1 |
| grapefruit, canned, unsweetened | 4 oz | 5 | 180 | 38 | 10 | 0.1 |
| grapefruit, canned, sweetened | 4 oz | 1 | 169 | 88 | 22 | 0.1 |
| grapefruit, canned, artificially sweetened | 4 oz | 1 |  | 45 | 9 | 0.5 |
| grapefruit, frozen, diluted, unsweetened | 4 oz | 1 | 213 | 51 | 12 | 0.1 |
| grapefruit, frozen, diluted, sweetened | 4 oz | 1 | 180 | 59 | 14 | 0.1 |
| grapefruit-orange, canned, unsweetened | 4 oz | 1 | 230 | 54 | 13 | 0.3 |
| grapefruit-orange, canned, sweetened | 4 oz | 1 | 230 | 63 | 15 | 0.1 |
| grapefruit-orange, frozen, diluted, unsweetened | 4 oz | <1 | 221 | 55 | 13 | 0.1 |
| grape juice, artificially sweetened | 4 oz | 2 |  | 71 | 18 | tr |
| grape juice, bottled | 4 oz | 3 | 145 | 83 | 21 | tr |
| grape juice, frozen, diluted | 4 oz | 1 | 43 | 66 | 17 | tr |
| lemon juice, canned, unsweetened | 1 tbsp | tr | 85 | 4 | 1 | tr |
| lemon juice, fresh | 1 tbsp | tr |  | 4 | 1 | tr |
| lemonade, frozen, diluted | 4 oz | tr | 20 | 55 | 14 | tr |
| lime juice, canned, unsweetened | 1 tbsp | tr | 16 | 4 | 1 | tr |

| | | | | | | |
|---|---|---|---|---|---|---|
| lime juice, fresh | 1 tbsp | tr | 16 | 4 | 1 | tr |
| limeade, frozen, diluted | 4 oz | tr | 16 | 51 | 14 | tr |
| orange juice, fresh | 4 oz | 1 | 249 | 56 | 13 | 0.3 |
| orange juice, canned, unsweetened | 4 oz | 1 | 249 | 60 | 14 | 0.3 |
| orange juice, canned, sweetened | 4 oz | 1 | 249 | 65 | 15 | 0.3 |
| orange juice, canned, artificially sweetened | 4 oz | 0.6 | | 55 | 13 | 0.3 |
| orange juice, frozen, diluted, unsweetened | 4 oz | 1 | 233 | 56 | 13 | 0.1 |
| orange-apricot juice, canned | 4 oz | tr | 118 | 63 | 16 | 0.1 |
| peach nectar, canned | 4 oz | 1 | 98 | 60 | 16 | tr |
| pear nectar, canned | 4 oz | 1 | 49 | 65 | 17 | 0.3 |
| pineapple juice, canned, unsweetened | 4 oz | 1 | 186 | 69 | 17 | 0.1 |
| pineapple juice, frozen, diluted, unsweetened | 4 oz | 1 | 170 | 65 | 16 | tr |
| prune juice, canned | 4 oz | 3 | 294 | 96 | 24 | 0.1 |
| tangerine juice, fresh | 4 oz | 1 | 223 | 54 | 13 | 0.3 |
| tangerine juice, canned, unsweetened | 4 oz | 1 | 223 | 54 | 13 | 0.3 |
| tangerine juice, frozen, diluted, unsweetened | 4 oz | 1 | 218 | 58 | 14 | 0.3 |
| tomato juice, canned | 4 oz | 250 | 284 | 24 | 5 | 0.1 |
| tomato cocktail | 4 oz | 250 | 276 | 26 | 6 | 0.1 |
| **Fruit Juices—Especially Prepared for Low-Sodium Diets** | | | | | | |
| Grape juice—Balanced | 4 oz | 2 | | 85 | 21 | 0 |
| Grapefruit juice—Featherweight | ½ cup | 5 | | 43 | 9 | 0 |
| Orange juice—Featherweight | ½ cup | 5 | | 53 | 12 | 0 |

| CATEGORY & FOOD | PORTION | SODIUM (mg) | POTASSIUM (mg) | CALORIES | CARBOHYDRATES (g) | FAT (g) |
|---|---|---|---|---|---|---|
| Pineapple Juice—Balanced | 4 oz | 5 | | 56 | 14 | 0.1 |
| Tomato juice—Arcadia | 4 oz | 13 | | 23 | 5 | 0 |
| Tomato Juice—Featherweight | 4 oz | 7 | | 23 | 5 | 0 |
| Tomato juice—S & W Nutradiet | 4 oz | 7 | | 23 | 5 | 0 |
| Tomato juice—Tillie Lewis | 4 oz | 17 | | | | |
| **Meats*** | | | | | | |
| bacon, raw | 1 slice | 71 | 16 | 156 | 0.2 | 16 |
| bacon, broiled | 1 slice | 76 | 17 | 48 | 0.2 | 4 |
| bacon, Canadian, raw | 1 slice | 440 | 90 | 65 | 0.1 | 4 |
| bacon Canadian, broiled | 1 slice | 442 | 91 | 65 | 3 | 4 |
| beef, brisket, cooked | 4 oz raw | 52 | 285 | 411 | 0 | 37 |
| beef, chipped | 4 oz | 4880 | 227 | 231 | 0 | 7 |
| beef, chuck, cooked | 4 oz | 53 | 439 | 371 | 0 | 32 |
| beef, club steak, broiled | 8 oz raw | 48 | 370 | 260 | 0 | 18 |
| beef, corned, canned | 1 slice | 268 | 17 | 60 | 0 | 3 |
| beef, corned, hash, canned | ½ cup | 997 | | 229 | 9 | 17 |
| beef, flank, cooked | 8 oz raw | 67 | 344 | 331 | 0 | 14 |
| beef, hamburger, broiled | 4 oz raw | 39 | 382 | 224 | 0 | 15 |

* Except for processed meats, no salt has been added in preparation.

| | | | | | | |
|---|---|---|---|---|---|---|
| beef, hash, cooked | ½ cup | 20 | | 145 | 14 | 5 |
| beef, heart, raw | ⅓ heart | 90 | 160 | 108 | 0.7 | 4 |
| beef, kidney, raw | 4 oz | 280 | 264 | 161 | 1 | 9 |
| beef, porterhouse, broiled | 8 oz raw | 52 | 398 | 242 | 0 | 15 |
| beef, rib roast, cooked | 8 oz raw | 57 | 438 | 302 | 0 | 7 |
| beef, rib steak, broiled | 8 oz raw | 50 | 388 | 246 | 0 | 17 |
| beef, bottom round, broiled | 8 oz raw | 51 | 552 | 271 | 0 | 11 |
| beef, top round, broiled | 8 oz raw | 46 | 547 | 254 | 0 | 6 |
| beef, round, pot roast | 8 oz raw | 43 | 309 | 188 | 0 | 9 |
| beef, short ribs, cooked | 8 oz raw | 39 | 297 | 290 | 0 | 24 |
| beef, sirloin, broiled | 8 oz raw | 57 | 545 | 260 | 0 | 14 |
| beef, sirloin tip, roast | 8 oz raw | 70 | 661 | 282 | 0 | 10 |
| beef, T-bone, broiled | 8 oz raw | 49 | 378 | 235 | 0 | 15 |
| beef, tenderloin, broiled | 8 oz raw | 60 | 576 | 296 | 0 | 17 |
| beef, tongue, cooked | 4 oz | 113 | 295 | 235 | 0.5 | 17 |
| ham, cured butt, cooked | 8 oz raw | 1036 | 478 | 246 | 0.4 | 13 |
| ham, cured butt, cooked | 1 slice | 518 | 239 | 123 | 0.2 | 7 |
| ham, cured shank, cooked | 8 oz raw | 682 | 314 | 185 | 0.2 | 11 |
| ham, boneless, canned | 4 oz | 1116 | | 189 | 0.5 | 11 |
| ham, fresh, cooked | 8 oz raw | 73 | 520 | 254 | 0 | 9 |
| ham, fresh, cooked | 1 slice | 37 | 260 | 126 | 0 | 5 |
| lamb, arm chop, cooked | 2 chops | 87 | 509 | 287 | 0 | 18 |
| lamb, blade chop, cooked | 1 chop | 72 | 422 | 260 | 0 | 17 |
| lamb, chop, broiled | 2 chops | 75 | 437 | 205 | 0 | 11 |

| CATEGORY & FOOD | PORTION | SODIUM (mg) | POTASSIUM (mg) | CALORIES | CARBOHYDRATES (g) | FAT (g) |
|---|---|---|---|---|---|---|
| lamb, rib chop, broiled | 2 chops | 68 | 398 | 238 | 0 | 0.7 |
| lamb, leg, roasted | 8 oz raw | 82 | 492 | 192 | 0 | 8 |
| liver, beef, raw | 4 oz | 98 | 371 | 155 | 7 | 4 |
| liver, calf's, raw | 4 oz | 150 | 498 | 161 | 5 | 6 |
| liver, chicken, simmered | 4 oz | 70 | 173 | 189 | 4 | 5 |
| liver, lamb, broiled | 4 oz | 97 | 378 | 298 | 3 | 14 |
| liver, turkey, simmered | 4 oz | 63 | 161 | 199 | 4 | 5 |
| pork, blade, cooked | 8 oz raw | 78 | 551 | 299 | 0 | 18 |
| pork, Boston butt, roasted | 8 oz raw | 83 | 592 | 328 | 0 | 22 |
| pork, loin chop, cooked | 8 oz raw | 69 | 667 | 419 | 0 | 30 |
| pork, picnic shoulder, roasted | 8 oz raw | 68 | 485 | 234 | 0 | 14.3 |
| pork, shoulder butt, cured, cooked | 4 oz | 765 | 368 | 440 | 0 | 38 |
| pork, sirloin, roasted | 8 oz raw | 52 | 481 | 215 | 0 | 10 |
| pork, spareribs, braised | 4 oz edible | 74 | 446 | 503 | 0 | 44 |
| pork, tenderloin, roasted | 4 oz | 63 | 582 | 273 | 0 | 14 |
| sweetbreads, beef, braised | 4 oz | 133 | 495 | 366 | 0 | 27 |
| veal, arm steak, cooked | 8 oz raw | 62 | 604 | 358 | 0 | 23 |
| veal, blade, cooked | 8 oz raw | 49 | 489 | 251 | 0 | 15 |
| veal, breast, stewed | 8 oz raw | 128 | 726 | 512 | 0 | 37 |
| veal, round cutlet, cooked | 8 oz raw | 61 | 597 | 313 | 0 | 17 |
| veal, loin chop, cooked | 8 oz raw | 54 | 384 | 514 | 0 | 44 |

| | | | | | | |
|---|---|---|---|---|---|---|
| veal, rib chop, cooked | 8 oz raw | 55 | 516 | 352 | 0 | 25 |
| veal, rump, roasted | 8 oz raw | 73 | 492 | 169 | 0 | 5 |
| veal, sirloin, roasted | 8 oz raw | 124 | 1114 | 172 | 0 | 6 |
| veal, sirloin steak, cooked | 8 oz raw | 52 | 512 | 355 | 0 | 23 |
| veal, stew meat | 8 oz raw | 99 | 561 | 395 | 0 | 29 |
| **Meats—Prepared or Processed** | | | | | | |
| bologna | 2 slices | 780 | 138 | 132 | 2 | 9 |
| chile con carne | 4 oz | 607 | 266 | 152 | 9 | 7 |
| frankfurter | 1 aver. | 542 | 108 | 124 | 1 | 10 |
| ham, smoked | 2 slices | 304 | | 60 | 0 | 3 |
| liverwurst spread | 2 oz | 508 | | 220 | 2 | 18 |
| luncheon meat | 2 slices | 745 | | 130 | 5 | 8 |
| pie, beef | 1 aver. dinner | 1008 | | 443 | 37 | 25 |
| pie, chicken meat | 1 aver. dinner | 863 | | 503 | 53 | 25 |
| pie, turkey meat | 1 aver. dinner | 864 | | 417 | 36 | 24 |
| salami | 2 slices | 510 | 266 | 152 | 9 | 7 |
| sausage, Braunschweiger liver | 2 slices | 636 | | 180 | 1 | 17 |
| sausage, pork | 4 oz | 846 | 160 | 342 | 0 | 30 |
| sausage, Vienna | 2 slices | 305 | | 90 | 1 | 8 |
| "TV" dinner, beef | 1 aver. dinner | 808 | | 349 | 25 | 14 |
| "TV" dinner, chicken | 1 aver. dinner | 1073 | | 542 | 42 | 28 |
| "TV" dinner, chopped sirloin | 1 aver. dinner | 1076 | | 483 | 25 | 29 |

| CATEGORY & FOOD | PORTION | SODIUM (mg) | POTASSIUM (mg) | CALORIES | CARBOHYDRATES (g) | FAT (g) |
|---|---|---|---|---|---|---|
| "TV" dinner, ham | 1 aver. dinner | 1173 | | 308 | 32 | 11 |
| "TV" dinner, loin of pork | 1 aver. dinner | 710 | | 414 | 40 | 18 |
| "TV" dinner, meat loaf | 1 aver. dinner | 1226 | | 369 | 29 | 18 |
| "TV" dinner, Swiss steak | 1 aver. dinner | 1072 | | 251 | 19 | 9 |
| **Meats and Other Dishes Especially Prepared for Low-Sodium Diets** | | | | | | |
| Beef ravioli—Featherweight | 8 oz | 100 | | 230 | 35 | 6 |
| Beef stew—Balanced | 8 oz | 71 | | 285 | 22 | 24 |
| Beef stew—Featherweight | 7¼ oz | 50 | | 210 | 24 | 8 |
| Boned chicken—Featherweight | 5 oz | 50 | | | | |
| Chicken stew—Featherweight | 7¼ oz | 30 | | 160 | 21 | 5 |
| Chile con carne w beans—Campbell's | 7¾ oz | 65 | | 340 | 33 | 16 |
| Chile with beans—Featherweight | 8 oz | 50 | | 360 | 31 | 19 |
| Stuffed dumplings w chicken—Featherweight | 8 oz | 95 | | 200 | 28 | 5 |
| Lamb stew—Featherweight | 7¼ oz | 45 | | 230 | 23 | 11 |
| Spaghetti with meatballs—Featherweight | 8 oz | 55 | | 200 | 24 | 8 |
| Spanish rice—Featherweight | 7¼ oz | 31 | | 140 | 28 | 1 |
| **Nuts and Nut Products*** | | | | | | |

* Prepared without salt unless otherwise indicated.

| | | | | | | |
|---|---|---|---|---|---|---|
| almonds, chocolate | 10 medium | 10 | 75 | 142 | 17 | 8 |
| almonds, dried, unblanched | 12-15 | 0.4 | 104 | 90 | 3 | 8 |
| almonds, dried, salted, unblanched | 12-15 | 24 | 106 | 93 | 3 | 9 |
| almond paste | 1 oz | 58 | 116 | 169 | 15 | 9 |
| almonds, unshelled | 1 cup | 1 | 276 | 238 | 8 | 22 |
| Brazil nuts, shelled | 4 medium | 0.2 | 100 | 97 | 2 | 10 |
| cashew nuts, roasted | 25 medium | 8 | 232 | 280 | 15 | 23 |
| chestnuts, fresh | 3 small | 0.3 | 62 | 29 | 6 | 0.2 |
| chestnuts, fresh, shelled | ½ cup | 2 | 410 | 191 | 42 | 2 |
| chestnuts, dried | ½ cup | 2 | | 189 | 39 | 2 |
| coconut, fresh meat | 1 piece | 3 | 116 | 54 | 2 | 5 |
| coconut, fresh, shredded | ½ cup | 8 | 374 | 175 | 7 | 17 |
| coconut, dried, shredded | ½ cup | 5 | 250 | 172 | 17 | 12 |
| dried seeds, unsalted, beans | ½ cup | 19 | 1196 | 340 | 61 | 2 |
| dried seeds, unsalted, beans, red | ½ cup | 10 | 984 | 343 | 62 | 2 |
| dried seeds, unsalted, chick-peas | ½ cup | 26 | 797 | 360 | 61 | 5 |
| dried seeds, unsalted, cowpeas | ½ cup | 35 | 1024 | 343 | 62 | 2 |
| dried seeds, unsalted, lentils | ½ cup | 30 | 790 | 340 | 60 | 1 |
| dried seeds, unsalted, lima beans | ½ cup | 3 | 1223 | 276 | 51 | 1 |
| dried seeds, unsalted, mung beans | 4 oz | 7 | 1175 | 389 | 69 | 1 |
| dried seeds, unsalted, peas, common | ½ cup | 35 | 1005 | 340 | 60 | 1 |
| dried seeds, unsalted, pigeon peas | 4 oz | 30 | 1121 | 391 | 73 | 2 |
| dried seeds, unsalted, soybeans | ½ cup | 5 | 1677 | 403 | 34 | 18 |

| CATEGORY & FOOD | PORTION | SODIUM (mg) | POTASSIUM (mg) | CALORIES | CARBOHYDRATES (g) | FAT (g) |
|---|---|---|---|---|---|---|
| dried seeds, unsalted, sunflower seeds | 1 oz | 9 | 263 | 160 | 6 | 14 |
| filberts or hazelnuts | 10-12 | 0.1 | 71 | 97 | 3 | 10 |
| litchi nuts, dried | 6 | 0.4 | 165 | 45 | 11 | 0.1 |
| mixed nuts, unsalted, shelled | 8-12 | 2 | 84 | 94 | 3 | 9 |
| peanuts, with skin, roasted | 1 oz | 0.6 | 211 | 163 | 6 | 13 |
| peanuts, without skin, salted, roasted | 1 oz | 131 | 200 | 162 | 5 | 13 |
| peanut butter | 1 tbsp | 75 | 123 | 95 | 2 | 9 |
| pecans, unsalted, shelled | 6 | tr | 63 | 104 | 2 | 11 |
| walnuts, English | 6-8 | 0.3 | 68 | 98 | 2 | 10 |
| **Nuts and Nut Products Especially Prepared for Low-Sodium Diets** | | | | | | |
| Almond butter, unsalted, raw—Hain | 1 tbsp | 0.8 | | 97 | 2 | 8 |
| Cashew butter, unsalted, raw—Hain | 1 tbsp | 3 | | 93 | 3 | 8 |
| Cashew butter, unsalted, roasted—Hain | 1 tbsp | 3 | | 93 | 4 | 7 |
| Mixed nuts, unsalted—Bazzini's | 1 oz | 8 | | | | |
| Peanut butter—Balanced | 1 tbsp | 3 | | | | |
| Peanut butter—Cellu | 1- oz | >5 | | 180 | 4 | 15 |
| Peanut butter—unsalted, raw—Hain | 1 tbsp | 2 | | 97 | 1 | 9 |
| Peanut butter—S & W | 1 tbsp | 8 | | 93 | 2 | 8 |

| | | | | | | |
|---|---|---|---|---|---|---|
| Peanut-sesame butter, unsalted, toasted—Hain | 1 tbsp | 2 | | 102 | 1 | 9 |
| Peanuts, unsalted—Flávor Tree | 1 oz | 3 | | 150 | 6 | 9 |
| Sesame butter, unsalted, raw—Hain | 1 tbsp | 3 | | | | |
| Soy beans, unsalted, roasted—Soy Town | 1 oz | 5 | | 140 | 5 | 10 |
| Soynuts, unsalted—Balanced | 1 oz | | | 130 | 6 | 7 |
| Sunflower butter, unsalted, raw—Hain | 1 tbsp | 1 | | 98 | 2 | 9 |
| **Poultry and Game** | | | | | | |
| chicken, broiler, raw, no bone | ¼ bird | 86 | 352 | 167 | 0 | 8 |
| chicken, broiled, no bone and skin | 4 oz | 75 | | 139 | 0 | 5 |
| chicken, broiler, fried, no bone | ¼ bird | 80 | 242 | 232 | 3 | 14 |
| chicken, roasted, dark meat, no skin | 4 oz | 100 | | 213 | 0 | 6 |
| chicken, roasted, white meat, no skin | 4 oz | 75 | | 213 | 0 | 5 |
| chicken, boned, canned w broth | 4 oz | 576 | | 176 | 2 | 10 |
| duck, domestic, raw | 4 oz | 94 | 326 | 373 | 0 | 33 |
| goose, domestic, raw | 4 oz | 98 | 480 | 405 | 0 | 36 |
| liver, chicken, simmered, chopped | ½ cup | 43 | | 115 | 3 | 3 |
| quail, raw | 4 oz | 46 | 200 | 192 | 0 | 8 |
| rabbit, domestic, raw | 4 oz | 46 | 440 | 182 | 0 | 7 |
| rabbit, domestic, stewed | 4 oz | 52 | | 240 | 0 | 12 |
| turkey, raw | 4 oz | 46 | 366 | 306 | 0 | 23 |
| turkey, roasted, dark meat, no skin | 4 oz | 112 | | 227 | 0 | 9 |

| CATEGORY & FOOD | PORTION | SODIUM (mg) | POTASSIUM (mg) | CALORIES | CARBOHYDRATES (g) | FAT (g) |
|---|---|---|---|---|---|---|
| turkey, roasted, white meat, no skin | 4 oz | 93 | | 200 | 0 | 5 |
| turkey, boned, canned w broth | 4 oz | 528 | | 176 | 0 | 8 |
| **Seasonings—Condiments** | | | | | | |
| catsup, tomato | 1 oz | 298 | 104 | 30 | 7 | 0.1 |
| chili sauce, tomato | 1 oz | 382 | 106 | 30 | 7 | 0.1 |
| mustard, brown | 1 tsp | 65 | 7 | 4 | 0.3 | 0.4 |
| pickles, dill, whole | 1 oz | 400 | 57 | 3 | 0.6 | 0.1 |
| pickles, sour | ½ large | 677 | | 5 | 1 | 0.1 |
| pickle relish, sweet | 1 oz | 303 | | 39 | 10 | 0.2 |
| **Seasonings—Condiments Especially Prepared for Low-Sodium Diets** | | | | | | |
| Catsup, tomato—Balanced | 1 tbsp | 5 | | 5 | 1 | 0 |
| Catsup, tomato—Featherweight | 1 oz | 5 | | 16 | 3 | 0 |
| Catsup, tomato—Tillie Lewis | 1 tbsp | <10 | | 8 | 2 | 0 |
| Chili sauce, tomato—Featherweight | 1 oz | 5 | | 16 | 3 | 0 |
| Cucumber relish—Featherweight | 1 oz | 5 | | 11 | 2 | 0 |
| Mustard, salad—Featherweight | 1 tsp | 0.5 | | | | |
| Pickles, kosher dill—Featherweight | 1 oz | 5 | | 5 | 0.9 | 0 |
| Pickles, sliced cucumber—Featherweight | 1 oz | 5 | | 12 | 3 | 0 |

| | | | | | | |
|---|---|---|---|---|---|---|
| Pickles, whole cucumber—Featherweight | 1 oz | 5 | | 12 | 3 | 0 |
| Pickles, whole dill—Featherweight | 1 oz | 5 | | 5 | 0.9 | 0 |
| **Seasonings—Salad Dressings** | | | | | | |
| blue cheese, Roquefort | 1 tbsp | 153 | 5 | 71 | 1 | 7 |
| blue cheese, Roquefort, low calorie | 1 tbsp | 155 | 5 | 11 | 0.6 | 0.8 |
| French dressing | 1 tbsp | 192 | 11 | 57 | 2 | 5 |
| French dressing, low calorie | 1 tbsp | 110 | 11 | 13 | 2 | 0.6 |
| Italian dressing | 1 tbsp | 293 | 2 | 77 | 1 | 8 |
| Italian dressing, low calorie | 1 tbsp | 110 | 2 | 7 | 0.4 | 0 |
| mayonnaise | 1 tbsp | 84 | 5 | 101 | 0.3 | 11 |
| mayonnaise type | 1 tbsp | 82 | 1 | 61 | 2 | 6 |
| mayonnaise type, low calorie | 1 tbsp | 17 | 1 | 19 | 0.7 | 2 |
| Russian dressing | 1 tbsp | 167 | | 55 | 7 | 3 |
| Russian dressing, low calorie | 1 tbsp | 160 | | 25 | 1 | 5 |
| Thousand Island | 1 tbsp | 98 | 16 | 70 | 2 | 7 |
| Thousand Island, low calorie | 1 tbsp | 98 | 16 | 25 | 2 | 2 |
| vinegar | 1 tbsp | 0.2 | 15 | 2 | 0.8 | 0 |
| **Seasonings—Salad Dressing Especially Prepared for Low-Sodium Diets** | | | | | | |
| Balanaise—Balanced | 1 tbsp | 6 | | | | |
| French dressing, unsalted—Arcadia | 1 tbsp | 3 | | 11 | | |
| French dressing unsalted—Balanced | 1 tbsp | 1 | | 11 | 0.6 | 0.9 |

| CATEGORY & FOOD | PORTION | SODIUM (mg) | POTASSIUM (mg) | CALORIES | CARBOHYDRATES (g) | FAT (g) |
|---|---|---|---|---|---|---|
| French, imitation, low-sodium—Cellu | 1 tbsp | 2 | | 60 | 1 | 6 |
| Herb dressing, unsalted—Hain | 1 tbsp | 1 | | | | |
| Italian dressing, unsalted—Arcadia | 1 tbsp | 0.3 | | 5 | | |
| Mayonnaise, unsalted—Arcadia | 1 tbsp | 7 | | | | |
| Mayonnaise, unsalted—Hain | 1 tbsp | 2 | | | | |
| Mayonnaise, eggless, unsalted—Hain | 1 tbsp | 1 | | 99 | 1 | 11 |
| Mayonnaise, unsalted—Melba | 1 tbsp | 5 | | 75 | | |
| Soyamaise, unsalted—Cellu | 1 tbsp | 6 | | 100 | 0 | 11 |
| 2 calories low-sodium—Featherweight | 1 tbsp | 10 | | 2 | 0 | 0 |
| Whipped dressing—Smithers | 1 tbsp | 6 | | 24 | | |
| **Seasonings—Salt** | | | | | | |
| salt, table | ½ tsp | 1165 | | | | |
| **Seasonings—Salt Substitutes Especially Prepared for Low-Sodium Diets** | | | | | | |
| Adolf's plain | ½ tsp | 0.3 | | | | |
| Adolf's seasoned | ½ tsp | 0.6 | | | | |
| Co-Salt | ½ tsp | 0.3 | | | | |
| Dia Mel | ½ tsp | 0.3 | | | | |
| Garlic salt substitute—Featherweight | ½ tsp | 2 | 1120 | | | |

| | | | | | | |
|---|---|---|---|---|---|---|
| K salt substitute—Featherweight | ½ tsp | 0.1 | 1092 | | | |
| Morton's plain | ½ tsp | <0.3 | | | | |
| Morton's seasoned | ½ tsp | <1.0 | | | | |
| McCormick plain | ½ tsp | <0.3 | | | | |
| McCormick seasoned | ½ tsp | <1.0 | | | | |
| Neocurtesal—Winthrop | ½ tsp | 0.3 | 1410 | | | |
| Nu-Salt—Sweet 'n Low | ½ tsp | <0.3 | | | | |
| Salt-It—Diamel | ½ tsp | 0.3 | | | | |
| Seasoned salt substitute—Featherweight | ½ tsp | 0.4 | 1092 | 3 | 0.1 | tr |
| **Seasonings—Sauces** | | | | | | |
| barbecue sauce | ¼ cup | 896 | | 105 | 25 | 1 |
| pizza sauce | ¼ cup | 266 | | 38 | 6 | 1 |
| seafood cocktail sauce | ¼ cup | 765 | | 70 | 17 | 1 |
| spaghetti sauce with meat | 2 tbsp | 244 | | 32 | 3 | 2 |
| spaghetti sauce with mushrooms | 2 tbsp | 248 | | 27 | 3 | 2 |
| tomato paste | 1 oz | 7 | 254 | 23 | 5 | 0.1 |
| tomato sauce | ¼ cup | 324 | | 20 | 8 | <1 |
| **Seasonings—Sauces Especially Prepared for Low-Sodium Diets** | | | | | | |
| Brown gravy—Van Winkle | 1 oz | 8 | | 5 | 1 | |
| Chicken gravy—Van Winkle | 1 oz | 22 | | 12 | 2 | |

| CATEGORY & FOOD | PORTION | SODIUM (mg) | POTASSIUM (mg) | CALORIES | CARBOHYDRATES (g) | FAT (g) |
|---|---|---|---|---|---|---|
| Spaghetti sauce, dietetic—Balanced | 1 oz | 17 | | 17 | 3 | 0.5 |
| Tomato paste—Balanced | 1 oz | 9 | | 27 | 6 | 0.1 |
| Tomato paste—Cellu | ¼ cup | 23 | | 56 | 13 | 0 |
| **Seasonings—Spices and Other Herb Seasonings** | | | | | | |
| allspice, ground | ¼ tsp | 2 | | | | |
| anise, seed | ¼ tsp | 0.2 | | | | |
| basil leaves | ¼ tsp | 0.2 | | | | |
| bay leaves | ¼ tsp | 0.4 | | | | |
| caraway, seed | ¼ tsp | 0.4 | | | | |
| cardamom, seed | ¼ tsp | 0.3 | | | | |
| cassia, cracked | ¼ tsp | 0.3 | | | | |
| celery flakes, dehydrated | ¼ tsp | 35 | | | | |
| celery seed | ¼ tsp | 2 | | | | |
| cinnamon, ground | ¼ tsp | 0.3 | | | | |
| cloves, ground | ¼ tsp | 0.3 | | | | |
| coriander, seed | ¼ tsp | 2 | | | | |
| cumin, ground | ¼ tsp | 0.2 | | | | |
| curry powder | ¼ tsp | 1 | | | | |
| dill seed | ¼ tsp | 0.3 | | | | |

| | | |
|---|---|---|
| fennel seed | ¼ tsp | 0.8 |
| fonugreek, seed | ¼ tsp | 1 |
| garlic powder | ¼ tsp | 0.3 |
| ginger, ground | ¼ tsp | 0.2 |
| Hickory smoked yeast (bacon flavor)—Sovex | 3 tsp | 2 |
| Italian seasoning—McCormick | ¼ tsp | 0.3 |
| mace, ground | ¼ tsp | 1.2 |
| marjoram, powdered | ¼ tsp | 0.5 |
| mint flakes, dehydrated | ¼ tsp | 0.6 |
| mustard, ground | ¼ tsp | 0.2 |
| nutmeg, ground | ¼ tsp | 0.4 |
| onion, minced, dehydrated | ¼ tsp | 0.7 |
| onion, powder | ¼ tsp | 1.4 |
| oregano, leaf | ¼ tsp | 0.5 |
| paprika, ground | ¼ tsp | 1.1 |
| parsley flakes, dehydrated | ¼ tsp | 7.2 |
| pepper, black, ground | ¼ tsp | 0.3 |
| pepper, red, ground | ¼ tsp | 0.4 |
| pepper, white, ground | ¼ tsp | 0.1 |
| Pickling spice—McCormick | ¼ tsp | 0.5 |
| poppy seed | ¼ tsp | 0.2 |
| Poultry seasoning—McCormick | ¼ tsp | 0.4 |
| rosemary, leaves | ¼ tsp | 0.7 |

| CATEGORY & FOOD | PORTION | SODIUM (mg) | POTAS-SIUM (mg) | CALO-RIES | CARBO-HYDRATES (g) | FAT (g) |
|---|---|---|---|---|---|---|
| saffron, Spanish | ¼ tsp | 0.4 | | | | |
| sage, rubbed | ¼ tsp | 0.2 | | | | |
| Salad herbs—Ehlers | ¼ tsp | 1.1 | | | | |
| savory, powdered | ¼ tsp | 0.3 | | | | |
| savory, rubbed | ¼ tsp | 0.8 | | | | |
| sesame, seed | ¼ tsp | 0.9 | | | | |
| Soup greens, dehydrated—McCormick | ¼ tsp | 1.3 | | | | |
| Spaghetti sauce seasoning—Van Winkle | for 2 oz of sauce | 0.4 | | 5 | 1 | tr |
| thyme, ground | ¼ tsp | 0.4 | | | | |
| thyme, powdered | ¼ tsp | 0.7 | | | | |
| turmeric, ground | ¼ tsp | 1 | | | | |
| Vegetable flakes, dehydrated—Ehlers | ¼ tsp | 2.6 | | | | |
| Vegetable flakes, dehydrated—McCormick | ¼ tsp | 2.7 | | | | |
| Vegit—Modern Products | ¼ tsp | 14 | | | | |
| **Snacks** | | | | | | |
| Bacon Rinds | 1 oz | 220 | | 145 | 0 | 8 |
| Cheese Flavored Flings | 1 oz (16) | 325 | 35 | 160 | 13 | 11 |
| Cheese Twists | 1 oz | 333 | | 155 | 15 | 10 |
| Chipsters, potato | 1 oz (57) | 685 | 165 | 130 | 18 | 6 |

| | | | | | | |
|---|---|---|---|---|---|---|
| Corn Chips | 1 oz | 220 | | 165 | 15 | 11 |
| Diggers corn snacks | 1 oz (36) | 310 | 30 | 160 | 17 | 9 |
| Doo Dads snacks | 1 oz (57) | 485 | 80 | 140 | 17 | 7 |
| Korkers corn twists | 1 oz (19) | 255 | 50 | 150 | 16 | 9 |
| Lil' Loaf snack sticks | 1 oz (10) | 340 | 70 | 140 | 18 | 7 |
| Onion Rings | 1 oz | 440 | | 135 | 20 | 6 |
| pizza, cheese, baked | 4 oz | 802 | 149 | 270 | 32 | 10 |
| pizza, sausage, baked | 4 oz | 833 | 192 | 267 | 34 | 11 |
| popcorn, oil and salt | 1 cup | 349 | | 82 | 11 | 4 |
| potato chips | 1 oz | 220 | 250 | 154 | 14 | 11 |
| Pretzels, Verithin, Mister Salty | 5 pretzels | 600 | 45 | 100 | 20 | 1 |
| soybeans, roasted | 1 oz | 228 | | 145 | 5 | 10 |
| Taco Tortilla chips | 1 oz | 242 | | 145 | 16 | 8 |
| Tortilla chips | 1 oz | 165 | | 150 | 18 | 8 |
| Twigs sesame, cheese flavored sticks | 1 oz (10) | 410 | 60 | 140 | 16 | 7 |
| **Snacks Especially Prepared for Low-Sodium Diets** | | | | | | |
| French onion sticks—Flavor Tree | 1 oz | 5 | | 149 | 14 | 9 |
| popcorn, no salt added | 1 cup | tr | | 54 | 11 | 0.7 |
| Potato Chips, unsalted—Health Maid | 1 oz | 16 | | | | |
| Potato Sticks, no salt added—Capitol Charter | 1 oz | 6 | | | | |
| Pretzels, low-sodium—Cellu | 2 pretzels | 3 | 26 | 14 | 3 | 0.2 |
| Sesame Sticks—Flavor Tree | 1 oz | 8 | | 162 | 13 | 11 |

| CATEGORY & FOOD | PORTION | SODIUM (mg) | POTASSIUM (mg) | CALORIES | CARBOHYDRATES (g) | FAT (g) |
|---|---|---|---|---|---|---|
| Soy beans, roasted, unsalted—Soy Town | 1 oz | 5 | | 140 | 5 | 10 |
| **Soups—Canned (Undiluted), Cubes, Packages** | | | | | | |
| Asparagus, cream—Campbell's | ½ can | 1222 | | 77 | 12 | 2 |
| Bean with bacon—Campbell's | ½ can | 1223 | | 218 | 28 | 7 |
| Bean with smoked pork—Heinz | ½ can | 1406 | | 211 | 24 | 8 |
| Bean, black—Campbell's | ½ can | 1402 | | 131 | 19 | 0.8 |
| Beef—Campbell's | ½ can | 1206 | | 137 | 12 | 3 |
| Beef, chunky—Campbell's | ½ can | 920 | | 210 | 21 | 7 |
| Beef broth—Campbell's | ½ can | 1177 | | 34 | 3 | 0 |
| Beef broth—Swanson | 8 oz | 760 | | 20 | 1 | 1 |
| Beef flavored, Cup-a-Broth—Lipton | 1 pkg | 899 | | 20 | 4 | 1 |
| Beef noodle—Campbell's | ½ can | 969 | | 88 | 11 | 3 |
| Beef noodle—Heinz | ½ can | 1310 | | 79 | 6 | 4 |
| Beef vegetable, barley—Heinz | ½ can | 1165 | | 87 | 10 | 2 |
| Bouillon cube, meat extract | 1 cube | 424 | 108 | 2 | 0 | 0.1 |
| Bouillon cube, vegetable extract | 1 cube | 245 | 138 | 8 | 2 | 0 |
| Celery, cream—Campbell's | ½ can | 1281 | | 97 | 11 | 5 |
| Celery, cream—Heinz | ½ can | 1092 | | 121 | 10 | 8 |
| Chicken, chunky—Campbell's | ½ can | 950 | | 200 | 20 | 7 |

| | | | | | |
|---|---|---|---|---|---|
| Chicken, cream—Campbell's | ½ can | 1192 | 118 | 9 | 7 |
| Chicken, cream—Heinz | ½ can | 1222 | 118 | 11 | 7 |
| Chicken broth—Campbell's | ½ can | 890 | 50 | 2 | 2 |
| Chicken broth—Swanson | 8 oz | 810 | 30 | 1 | 2 |
| Chicken flavored, Cup-a-Broth—Lipton's | 1 pkg | 788 | 25 | 4 | 1 |
| Chicken gumbo—Campbell's | ½ can | 1341 | 69 | 11 | 2 |
| Chicken gumbo—Heinz | ½ can | 1022 | 69 | 7 | 2 |
| Chicken noodle—Campbell's | ½ can | 1133 | 76 | 10 | 2 |
| Chicken noodle—Heinz | ½ can | 1304 | 79 | 9 | 3 |
| Chicken rice—Campbell's | ½ can | 1138 | 48 | 6 | 0.8 |
| Chicken rice—Heinz | ½ can | 1154 | 67 | 8 | 2 |
| Chicken rice—Lipton's | 1 cup | 948 | 65 | 8 | 2 |
| Chicken with rice, chunky—Campbell's | ½ can | 1005 | 160 | 16 | 4 |
| Chicken vegetable—Campbell's | ½ can | 1247 | 97 | 11 | 4 |
| Chicken vegetable—Heinz | ½ can | 1326 | 91 | 12 | 2 |
| Chicken vegetable—Lipton's | 1 cup | 1160 | 75 | 10 | 2 |
| Clam chowder, chunky—Campbell's | ½ can | 1130 | 160 | 15 | 3 |
| Clam chowder, Manhattan—Campbell's | ½ can | 1109 | 98 | 14 | 3 |
| Clam chowder, Manhattan—Heinz | ½ can | 1241 | 89 | 12 | 3 |
| Consommé, beef—Campbell's | ½ can | 765 | 43 | 4 | 0 |
| Consommé, chicken—Heinz | ½ can | 900 | 27 | 2 | 0.2 |
| Green pea—Campbell's | ½ can | 1212 | 170 | 27 | 3 |
| Green pea—Heinz | ½ can | 1108 | 164 | 29 | 3 |

| CATEGORY & FOOD | PORTION | SODIUM (mg) | POTASSIUM (mg) | CALORIES | CARBOHYDRATES (g) | FAT (g) |
|---|---|---|---|---|---|---|
| Green pea—Lipton's | 1 cup | 1078 | | 140 | 23 | 2 |
| Green pea, Cup-a-Soup—Lipton's | 1 pkg | 694 | | 130 | 22 | 2 |
| Gumbo, creole—Heinz | ½ can | 2078 | | 87 | 14 | 3 |
| Minestrone—Campbell's | ½ can | 1274 | | 124 | 14 | 4 |
| Minestrone—Heinz | ½ can | 1252 | | 130 | 20 | 4 |
| Mushroom, cream—Campbell's | ½ can | 1162 | | 169 | 13 | 12 |
| Mushroom, cream—Heinz | ½ can | 1210 | | 164 | 11 | 12 |
| Mushroom, cream, Cup-a-Soup—Lipton's | 1 pkg | 527 | | 90 | 10 | 5 |
| Mushroom with beef—Lipton's | 1 cup | 929 | | 40 | 6 | 1 |
| Noodle, beef flavor with veg—Lipton's | 1 cup | 1258 | | 65 | 11 | 2 |
| Noodle w beef flav, Cup-a-Soup—Lipton's | 1 pkg | 892 | | 35 | 7 | 1 |
| Noodle, w chicken flav, Cup-a-Soup—Lipton's | 1 pkg | 931 | | 40 | 6 | 1 |
| Noodle with chicken broth—Lipton's | 1 cup | 888 | | 55 | 7 | 2 |
| Noodle with diced chicken—Lipton's | 1 cup | 971 | | 70 | 9 | 2 |
| Noodle w chicken, Cup-a-Soup—Lipton's | 1 pkg | 989 | | 45 | 6 | 1 |
| Onion—Campbell's | ½ can | 1304 | | 78 | 6 | 3 |
| Onion—Lipton's | 1 cup | 872 | | 35 | 6 | 1 |
| Onion, Cup-a-Soup—Lipton's | 1 pkg | 920 | | 30 | 6 | 1 |
| Pepper pot—Campbell's | ½ can | 1560 | | 131 | 12 | 5 |
| Scotch broth—Campbell's | ½ can | 1525 | | 114 | 13 | 4 |

| | | | | | |
|---|---|---|---|---|---|
| Split pea—Heinz | ½ can | 1171 | 179 | 25 | 4 |
| Split pea with ham, chunky—Campbell's | ½ can | 1055 | 220 | 30 | 5 |
| Tomato—Campbell's | ½ can | 1207 | 109 | 18 | 3 |
| Tomato—Heinz | ½ can | 1184 | 116 | 19 | 3 |
| Tomato, Cup-a-Soup—Lipton's | 1 pkg | 670 | 80 | 18 | 1 |
| Tomato, rice—Campbell's | ½ can | 915 | 90 | 19 | 2 |
| Tomato vegetable—Lipton's | 1 cup | 1304 | 70 | 12 | 2 |
| Turkey noodle—Campbell's | ½ can | 1132 | 88 | 11 | 3 |
| Turkey noodle—Heinz | ½ can | 1350 | 103 | 10 | 4 |
| Turkey noodle—Lipton's | 1 cup | 933 | 60 | 8 | 1 |
| Turtle, genuine—Heinz | ½ can | 1574 | 64 | 10 | 0.8 |
| Vegetable—Campbell's | ½ can | 854 | 87 | 16 | 2 |
| Vegetable, Cup-a-Soup—Lipton's | 1 pkg | 1065 | 45 | 8 | 1 |
| Vegetable, beef—Campbell's | ½ can | 1230 | 96 | 9 | 3 |
| Vegetable, beef—Heinz | ½ can | 1374 | 96 | 13 | 3 |
| Vegetarian vegetable—Campbell's | ½ can | 654 | 95 | 16 | 2 |
| Vegetarian vegetable—Heinz | ½ can | 1204 | 95 | 15 | 3 |

**Soups—Frozen (Does Not Include Sodium Value of Milk)**

| | | | | | |
|---|---|---|---|---|---|
| Clam chowder, New England—Campbell's | ⅓ can | 894 | 173 | 14 | 10 |
| Green pea with ham—Campbell's | ⅓ can | 745 | 99 | 14 | 2 |
| Oyster stew—Campbell's | ⅓ can | 645 | 97 | 7 | 6 |
| Potato, cream—Campbell's | ⅓ can | 951 | 87 | 10 | 3 |

| CATEGORY & FOOD | PORTION | SODIUM (mg) | POTASSIUM (mg) | CALORIES | CARBOHYDRATES (g) | FAT (g) |
|---|---|---|---|---|---|---|
| Shrimp, cream—Campbell's | ⅓ can | 813 | | 126 | 7 | 9 |
| **Soups Especially Prepared for Low-Sodium Diets** | | | | | | |
| Beef bouillon cubes—Featherweight | 1 cube | 10 | | 12 | 2 | 1 |
| Beef soup base—Featherweight | 5.3 gr | 7 | | 20 | 3 | 0.8 |
| Borsch, unsalted—Mother's | 8 oz | 37 | | | | |
| Chicken bouillon cubes—Featherweight | 1 cube | 5 | | 12 | 2 | 1 |
| Chicken broth—Featherweight | ¾ cup | 51 | | | | |
| Chicken noodle—Featherweight | 4 oz | 10 | | 60 | 7 | 2 |
| Chicken noodle—Tillie Lewis | 4 oz | 23 | | | | |
| Chicken soup base—Featherweight | 5.3 gr | 1 | | 25 | 4 | 1 |
| Cream of mushroom—Balanced | 4 oz | 30 | | 40 | 5 | 2 |
| Cream of mushroom—Campbell's | 4 oz | 11 | 39 | 72 | 6 | 5 |
| Cream of mushroom—Featherweight | 4 oz | 30 | | 50 | 9 | 0.5 |
| Green pea—Balanced | 4 oz | 13 | | 49 | 10 | 0.1 |
| Green pea—Campbell's | 4 oz | 21 | 70 | 75 | 12 | 2 |
| Green pea—Featherweight | 4 oz | 15 | | 11 | 18 | 1 |
| Tomato—Campbell's | 4 oz | 17 | 168 | 55 | 10 | 1 |
| Tomato—Featherweight | 4 oz | 15 | | 11 | 18 | 1 |
| Tomato—Tillie Lewis | 4 oz | 17 | | 32 | 5 | 0.7 |

| | | | | | | |
|---|---|---|---|---|---|---|
| Tomato—Van Winkle | 5 oz | 1 | | 25 | 12 | |
| Tomato with rice—Balanced | 4 oz | 18 | | 37 | 7 | 0.5 |
| Turkey noodle—Campbell's | 4 oz | 22 | 27 | 33 | 4 | 1 |
| Vegetable—Arcadia | 4 oz | 32 | | 29 | | |
| Vegetable—Campbell's | 4 oz | 22 | 94 | 44 | 8 | 11 |
| Vegetable—Tillie Lewis | 4 oz | 20 | | | | |
| Vegetable beef—Campbell's | 4 oz | 25 | 80 | 44 | 4 | 2 |
| Vegetable beef—Featherweight | 4 oz | 20 | | 80 | 11 | 3 |
| Vegetable bouillon—Morga | 1 cube | 37 | | | | |
| **Sweets—Candies** | | | | | | |
| Chuckles fruit flavored jellies | 1 piece | <10 | | | | |
| Chuckles jelly rings | 1 piece | <50 | | | | |
| Chuckles Jujubes | 1 piece | <50 | | | | |
| Chuckles marshmallow eggs | 1 piece | <10 | | | | |
| Chuckles nougat centers | 1 piece | <50 | | | | |
| Chuckles orange slices | 1 piece | <50 | | | | |
| Chuckles small eggs | 1 piece | <50 | | | | |
| Chuckles spearmint leaves | 1 piece | <50 | | | | |
| Chuckles spice slices | 1 piece | <50 | | | | |
| Chuckles spice sticks and drops | 1 piece | <50 | | | | |
| Hershey's chocolate almond bar | 1 oz | 10 | 75 | 142 | 17 | 8 |
| Hershey's milk chocolate bar | 1 oz | 30 | 105 | 152 | 16 | 10 |

| CATEGORY & FOOD | PORTION | SODIUM (mg) | POTASSIUM (mg) | CALORIES | CARBOHYDRATES (g) | FAT (g) |
|---|---|---|---|---|---|---|
| Hershey's milk chocolate kisses | 1 piece | 4 | 15 | 21 | 2 | 1 |
| Hershey's milk chocolate covered almonds | 1 oz | 10 | 75 | 142 | 17 | 8 |
| Hershey's Mr. Goodbar | 1 oz | 20 | 120 | 153 | 13 | 10 |
| Hershey's semi-sweet chocolate bar | 1 oz | 5 | 95 | 147 | 18 | 9 |
| Milky Way | 1 bar | 165 | 112 | 284 | 58 | 5 |
| Nabisco butterscotch skimmers | 1 piece | <50 | | | | |
| Nabisco chocolate covered cherries | 1 piece | <10 | | | | |
| Nabisco Jamaica mints | 1 piece | <50 | | | | |
| Nabisco milk chocolate stars | 1 piece | <50 | | | | |
| Nabisco mint wafers | 1 piece | <10 | | | | |
| Nabisco peppermint patties | 1 piece | <10 | | | | |
| Pom Poms, caramels | 1 piece | <50 | | | | |
| Sugar Babies caramel candies | 1 piece | <50 | | | | |
| Sugar Daddy caramel nuggets | 1 piece | <50 | | | | |
| Sugar Daddy caramel pop | 1 piece | <50 | | | | |
| Whirligigs caramel | 1 piece | <50 | | | | |
| **Sweets—Candies Especially Prepared for Low-Sodium Diets** | | | | | | |
| Chocolate bar, almond 3/4 oz—Estee | 1 bar | 33 | | 127 | 10 | 9 |
| Chocolate bar, almond 1 oz—Estee | 1 section | 4 | | 14 | 1 | 1 |

| | | | | | | |
|---|---|---|---|---|---|---|
| Chocolate bar, almond 3 oz—Estee | 1 section | 22 | | 80 | 6 | 6 |
| Chocolate bar, bittersweet 3/4 oz—Estee | 1 bar | 22 | | 127 | 11 | 9 |
| Chocolate bar, bittersweet 2 oz—Estee | 1 section | 2 | | 14 | 1 | 1 |
| Chocolate bar, bittersweet 3 oz—Estee | 1 section | 15 | | 80 | 7 | 6 |
| Chocolate bar, milk 3/4 oz—Estee | 1 bar | 31 | | 127 | 9 | 9 |
| Chocolate bar, milk 2 oz—Estee | 1 section | 3 | | 14 | 1 | 1 |
| Chocolate bar, milk 3 oz—Estee | 1 section | 21 | | 80 | 6 | 6 |
| Chocolate bar, fruit and nut 3 oz—Estee | 1 section | 26 | | 80 | 6 | 6 |
| Chocolate bar, white 3 oz—Estee | 1 section | 23 | | 80 | 7 | 5 |
| Chocolate covered almonds—Estee | 1 nut | 4 | | 17 | | |
| Chocolate covered peanuts—Estee | 1 nut | 1 | | 8 | | |
| Chocolate peanut butter cups—Estee | 1 cup | 8 | | 45 | | |
| Chocolate TV mix—Estee | 1 piece | 1 | | 9 | | |
| Gumdrops, assorted—Estee | 1 drop | 0.1 | | 3 | 0.8 | tr |
| Gumdrops, licorice—Estee | 1 drop | 0.1 | | 3 | 0.6 | tr |
| Hard candies, assorted peppermint—Estee | 1 candy | 0.2 | | 13 | | |
| Hard candies, cough, licorice—Estee | 1 candy | 0.2 | | 13 | | |
| Hard candies, coffee—Estee | 1 candy | 0.2 | | 13 | | |
| Mints, fruit flavored—Estee | 1 mint | 0.1 | | 4 | | |
| Mints, peppermint, spearmint—Estee | 1 mint | 0.1 | | 4 | | |
| Raisins, chocolate covered—Estee | 1 raisin | 1.1 | | 5 | | |

| CATEGORY & FOOD | PORTION | SODIUM (mg) | POTASSIUM (mg) | CALORIES | CARBOHYDRATES (g) | FAT (g) |
|---|---|---|---|---|---|---|
| **Sweets—Jams and Jellies** | | | | | | |
| apple butter, canned | 1 tbsp | 0.4 | 50 | 37 | 9 | 0.2 |
| assorted jams, commercial | 1 tbsp | 2 | 18 | 54 | 14 | tr |
| assorted jellies, commercial | 1 tbsp | 3 | 15 | 55 | 14 | tr |
| chutney, apple | 1 tbsp | 34 | 43 | 41 | 10 | tr |
| chutney, tomato | 1 tbsp | 26 | 56 | 31 | 8 | |
| marmalade, citrus | 1 tbsp | 3 | 7 | 51 | 14 | tr |
| **Sweets—Jams and Jellies Especially Prepared for Low-Sodium Diet** | | | | | | |
| Apple spread—Balanced | 1 tbsp | 0.5 | | 28 | 7 | tr |
| **Sweets—Sugars and Syrups** | | | | | | |
| honey, strained | 1 tbsp | 1 | 10 | 61 | 17 | 0 |
| molasses | 1 tbsp | 16 | 300 | 50 | 13 | 0 |
| sugar, brown | 1 tbsp | 3 | 32 | 52 | 13 | 0 |
| sugar, white | 1 tbsp | tr | tr | 46 | 12 | 0 |
| Syrup, chocolate flavored—Hershey's | 1 tbsp | 11 | 39 | 49 | 12 | 0.2 |
| Syrup, vitamin fortified—Hershey's | 1 tbsp | 1 | 65 | 55 | 13 | 0.3 |
| Syrup, chocolate fudge topping—Hershey's | 1 tbsp | 82 | 46 | 68 | 11 | 3 |

| | | | | | | |
|---|---|---|---|---|---|---|
| Sweet 'n Low, sugar substitute | 1 pkg | 3 | | 3 | .9 | |
| **Sweets—Sugars Especially Prepared for Low-Sodium Diet** | | | | | | |
| Zero Cal—Sweet 'n Low | 1 pkg | 0 | | 0 | 0 | 0 |
| **Vegetables** | | | | | | |
| artichoke, raw | 1 large | 86 | 860 | 88 | 21 | 0.4 |
| artichoke, cooked, edible parts | 1 large | 30 | 301 | 44 | 10 | 0.2 |
| artichoke hearts, frozen | 3 oz | 40 | 211 | 20 | 5 | 0 |
| asparagus, raw | 6 spears | 2 | 278 | 26 | 5 | 0.2 |
| asparagus, cooked | ½ cup | 0.8 | 137 | 15 | 3 | 0.1 |
| asparagus, green, canned | 6 spears | 271 | 191 | 21 | 3 | 0.3 |
| asparagus, white, canned | 6 spears | 271 | 161 | 21 | 4 | 0.3 |
| asparagus, frozen | 6 spears | 2 | 239 | 23 | 4 | 0.2 |
| beans, baby butter, frozen | 3 oz | 155 | 485 | 118 | 22 | 0 |
| beans, common white, dry, raw | ½ cup | 19 | 1196 | 340 | 61 | 2 |
| beans, common white, dry, cooked | ½ cup | 7 | 416 | 118 | 21 | 0.6 |
| beans, with pork and tomato—canned | ½ cup | 579 | 263 | 152 | 24 | 3 |
| beans, with pork and molasses—canned | ½ cup | 475 | | 188 | 26 | 6 |
| beans, without pork—canned | ½ cup | 422 | 335 | 150 | 29 | 0.6 |
| beans, green, raw | ½ cup | 7 | 243 | 32 | 7 | 0.2 |
| beans, green, cooked | ½ cup | 5 | 189 | 31 | 7 | 0.2 |
| beans, green, canned | ½ cup | 270 | 104 | 20 | 5 | 0.1 |

| CATEGORY & FOOD | PORTION | SODIUM (mg) | POTASSIUM (mg) | CALORIES | CARBOHYDRATES (g) | FAT (g) |
|---|---|---|---|---|---|---|
| beans, green, cut, frozen | 3 oz | 2 | 166 | 25 | 5 | 0 |
| beans, green, French style, frozen | 3 oz | 2 | 148 | 30 | 6 | 0 |
| beans, green, Italian, frozen | 3 oz | 4 | 217 | 30 | 6 | 0 |
| beans, green, whole, frozen | 3 oz | 3 | 105 | 25 | 5 | 0 |
| beans, lima, baby, frozen | 3 oz | 98 | 320 | 109 | 18 | 1 |
| beans, lima, green, raw | 4 tbsp | 2 | 650 | 123 | 22 | 0.5 |
| beans, lima, green, cooked | ½ cup | 0.8 | 338 | 89 | 16 | 0.4 |
| beans, lima, green, canned | ½ cup | 271 | 255 | 110 | 21 | 0.3 |
| beans, lima, tiny, frozen | 3 oz | 98 | 320 | 109 | 18 | 1 |
| beans, lima, dry seeds, raw | ½ cup | 4 | 1529 | 345 | 64 | 2 |
| beans, lima, dry seeds, cooked | ½ cup | 2 | 563 | 127 | 24 | 0.6 |
| beans, mung dry, raw | 3 oz | 5 | 881 | 291 | 52 | 1 |
| beans, mung sprouted seeds, raw | 3 oz | 4 | 191 | 30 | 6 | 0.2 |
| beans, mung sprouted seeds, cooked | 3 oz | 3 | 134 | 24 | 4 | 0.2 |
| beans, pinto, dry, raw | ½ cup | 10 | 984 | 349 | 64 | 1 |
| beans, red kidney, dry, raw | ½ cup | 10 | 984 | 343 | 62 | 2 |
| beans, red kidney, dry, cooked | ½ cup | 4 | 425 | 148 | 27 | 0.6 |
| beans, red kidney, dry, canned | ½ cup | 4 | 330 | 113 | 21 | 0.5 |
| beans, wax, raw | ½ cup | 4 | 122 | 14 | 4 | 0.1 |
| beans, wax, cooked | ½ cup | 2 | 76 | 11 | 2 | 0.1 |
| beans, wax, canned | ½ cup | 236 | 95 | 24 | 5 | 0.3 |

| | | | | | | |
|---|---|---|---|---|---|---|
| beans, wax, frozen | 3 oz | 2 | 228 | 30 | 4 | 0 |
| beets, red, raw | 1 (2") | 30 | 168 | 22 | 5 | 0.1 |
| beets, red, diced, cooked | ½ cup | 36 | 172 | 27 | 6 | 0.1 |
| beets, red, diced, canned | ½ cup | 196 | 138 | 31 | 7 | 0.1 |
| beet greens, cooked | ½ cup | 76 | 332 | 18 | 3 | 0.2 |
| broccoli, flower stalk, raw | 1 stalk | 15 | 382 | 32 | 6 | 0.3 |
| broccoli, flower stalk, cooked | 1 stalk | 10 | 267 | 26 | 5 | 0.3 |
| broccoli, baby spears, frozen | 3 oz | 13 | 223 | 23 | 4 | 0 |
| broccoli, spears, frozen | 3 oz | 9 | 202 | 23 | 4 | 0 |
| broccoli, spears, chopped, frozen | 3 oz | 13 | 186 | 23 | 4 | 0 |
| brussels sprouts, raw | 9 sprouts | 14 | 390 | 45 | 8 | 0.4 |
| brussels sprouts, cooked | ½ cup | 8 | 205 | 27 | 5 | 0.3 |
| brussels sprouts, baby, frozen | 3 oz | 5 | 347 | 32 | 5 | 0 |
| brussels sprouts, frozen | 3 oz | 4 | 306 | 27 | 5 | 0 |
| cabbage, headed, shredded, raw | 1 cup | 20 | 233 | 24 | 5 | 0.2 |
| cabbage, cooked | ½ cup | 12 | 136 | 17 | 4 | 0.2 |
| cabbage, Chinese, shredded, raw | 1 cup | 10 | 112 | 6 | 2 | tr |
| cabbage, red, shredded, raw | 1 cup | 26 | 268 | 31 | 7 | 0.2 |
| cabbage, savoy, shredded, raw | 1 cup | 11 | 135 | 12 | 2 | 0.1 |
| cabbage, spoon, raw | 3 oz | 22 | 262 | 14 | 2 | 0.2 |
| cabbage, spoon, cooked | 3 oz | 15 | 183 | 12 | 2 | 0.2 |
| carrots, raw | 1 large | 47 | 341 | 42 | 10 | 0.2 |
| carrots, cooked | ½ cup | 25 | 167 | 23 | 5 | 0.1 |
| carrots, canned | ½ cup | 177 | 90 | 23 | 5 | 0.2 |

| CATEGORY & FOOD | PORTION | SODIUM (mg) | POTASSIUM (mg) | CALORIES | CARBOHYDRATES (g) | FAT (g) |
|---|---|---|---|---|---|---|
| cauliflower, raw | 1 cup | 6 | 118 | 13 | 2 | 0.1 |
| cauliflower, cooked | ½ cup | 10 | 118 | 10 | 2 | 0.1 |
| cauliflower, frozen | 3 oz | 11 | 202 | 23 | 4 | 0 |
| celeriac root, raw | 5 roots | 100 | 300 | 40 | 9 | 0.3 |
| celery, raw | 1 stalk | 50 | 136 | 8 | 2 | tr |
| celery, diced, raw | 1 cup | 126 | 341 | 17 | 4 | 0.1 |
| celery, diced, cooked | ½ cup | 55 | 149 | 9 | 2 | 0.1 |
| chard, leaves, raw | ½ cup cooked | 123 | 458 | 21 | 4 | 0.3 |
| chard, leaves, cooked | ½ cup | 72 | 268 | 15 | 3 | 0.2 |
| chard, chayote, raw | 1 med | 5 | 102 | 28 | 7 | 0.1 |
| chick-peas, dried | ½ cup | 26 | 797 | 360 | 61 | 5 |
| chicory, raw | 10 leaves | 2 | 46 | 4 | 0.8 | tr |
| collards, raw | ½ cup | 43 | 401 | 40 | 7 | 0.7 |
| collards, cooked | ½ cup | 25 | 234 | 29 | 5 | 0.6 |
| collards, frozen | 3 oz | 41 | 217 | 27 | 4 | 0 |
| corn, kernels, cooked | 1 ear | tr | 196 | 100 | 21 | 1 |
| corn, kernels, canned | ½ cup | 295 | 121 | 83 | 20 | 0.8 |
| corn on the cob, raw | 1 ear | tr | 280 | 96 | 22 | 1 |
| corn on the cob, frozen | 1 ear | 3 | 425 | 130 | 28 | 1 |
| corn on the cob, little ears, frozen | 1 ear | 2 | 255 | 70 | 15 | 1 |
| corn, whole kernels, frozen | 3 oz | 2 | 174 | 64 | 20 | 0 |

| | | | | | | |
|---|---|---|---|---|---|---|
| cowpeas, (also blackeyes), raw | ½ cup | 2 | 406 | 95 | 16 | 0.6 |
| cowpeas, cooked | ½ cup | 1 | 303 | 86 | 15 | 0.6 |
| cowpeas, canned | ½ cup | 236 | 352 | 70 | 12 | 0.3 |
| cowpeas (blackeye), cooked, frozen | 3 oz | 33 | 289 | 111 | 20 | 0.3 |
| cress, raw | 6 sprigs | 1 | 61 | 3 | 0.6 | 0.1 |
| cress, cooked | 3 oz | 7 | 303 | 20 | 3 | 0.5 |
| cress, cooked | ½ cup | 6 | 243 | 15 | 3 | 0.5 |
| cucumber, raw | ½ med | 3 | 80 | 8 | 2 | 0.1 |
| dandelion greens, raw | ½ cup | 76 | 397 | 45 | 9 | 0.7 |
| dandelion greens, cooked | ½ cup | 44 | 232 | 33 | 6 | 0.6 |
| dock, raw | ½ cup | 5 | 338 | 28 | 6 | 0.3 |
| dock, cooked | ½ cup | 3 | 198 | 19 | 4 | 0.2 |
| eggplant, diced, raw | ½ cup | 2 | 214 | 25 | 6 | 0.2 |
| eggplant, diced, cooked | ½ cup | 1 | 150 | 19 | 4 | 0.2 |
| endive, raw | 10 leaves | 7 | 147 | 10 | 2 | 0.1 |
| escarole, raw | 2 lg leaves | 7 | 147 | 10 | 2 | 0.1 |
| ginger root, fresh | 2 oz | 3 | 151 | 28 | 5 | 0.2 |
| kale, raw | ½ cup | 50 | 212 | 25 | 4 | 0.5 |
| kale, cooked | ½ cup | 29 | 147 | 19 | 3 | 0.5 |
| kale, chopped, frozen | 3 oz | 43 | 191 | 55 | 10 | 0 |
| kohlrabi, diced, raw | ½ cup | 6 | 279 | 22 | 5 | 0.1 |
| kohlrabi, cooked | ½ cup | 5 | 195 | 18 | 4 | 0.1 |
| leeks, raw | 3-4 | 5 | 347 | 52 | 11 | 0.3 |
| lentils, dry, raw | ½ cup | 30 | 790 | 340 | 60 | 1 |

| CATEGORY & FOOD | PORTION | SODIUM (mg) | POTASSIUM (mg) | CALORIES | CARBOHYDRATES (g) | FAT (g) |
|---|---|---|---|---|---|---|
| lettuce, Boston, raw | 2 med leaves | 1 | | 2 | <1 | <1 |
| lettuce, Iceberg, raw | ¼ med head | 12 | 352 | 18 | 4 | <1 |
| lettuce, romaine, raw | 3 long leaves | 9 | 264 | 14 | 3 | 0.2 |
| mixed vegetables, frozen | 3 oz | 43 | 191 | 55 | 10 | 0 |
| mushrooms, raw | 4 large | 15 | 414 | 28 | 4 | 0.5 |
| mushrooms, canned | ½ cup | 400 | 197 | 17 | 2 | 0.1 |
| mustard greens, raw | ½ cup | 32 | 377 | 31 | 6 | 0.5 |
| mustard greens, cooked | ½ cup | 18 | 220 | 23 | 4 | 0.4 |
| mustard greens, chopped, frozen | 3 oz | 25 | 145 | 16 | 3 | 0 |
| New Zealand spinach, raw | 3 oz | 136 | 681 | 16 | 3 | 0.3 |
| New Zealand spinach, cooked | 3 oz | 79 | 397 | 11 | 2 | 0.2 |
| okra, raw | 8-9 pods | 3 | 249 | 36 | 8 | 0.3 |
| okra, cooked | 8-9 pods | 2 | 174 | 29 | 6 | 0.3 |
| okra, cut, frozen | 3 oz | 3 | 161 | 23 | 5 | 0 |
| okra, whole, frozen | 3 oz | 2 | 150 | 32 | 6 | 0 |
| onions, mature, raw | 1 med | 10 | 157 | 38 | 9 | 0.1 |
| onions, chopped, raw | 1 tbsp | 1 | 16 | 4 | 0.9 | tr |
| onions, cooked | ½ cup | 7 | 110 | 29 | 7 | 0.1 |
| onions, dehydrated flakes | ½ oz | 13 | 198 | 50 | 12 | 0.2 |
| onions, chopped, frozen | 1 oz | 7 | 141 | 8 | 2 | 0 |
| onions, small whole, frozen | 3 oz | 8 | 119 | 30 | 7 | 0 |

| | | | | | | |
|---|---|---|---|---|---|---|
| onions, (scallions), raw | 1 med | 1 | 46 | 9 | 2 | tr |
| parsley, raw | 1 oz | 13 | 208 | 13 | 2 | 0.2 |
| parsley, chopped, raw | 1 tbsp | 4 | 73 | 4 | 0.8 | tr |
| parsnips, raw | 1 large | 24 | 1082 | 152 | 35 | 1 |
| parsnips, cooked | ½ cup | 8 | 379 | 66 | 15 | 0.5 |
| peas, green, shelled, raw | ½ cup | 1 | 211 | 56 | 10 | 0.3 |
| peas, green, cooked | ½ cup | 0.8 | 147 | 53 | 9 | 0.3 |
| peas, green, drained, canned | ½ cup | 177 | 72 | 66 | 13 | 0.3 |
| peas, green, frozen | 3 oz | 99 | 149 | 64 | 10 | 0 |
| peas, tender tiny, frozen | 3 oz | 115 | 124 | 55 | 8 | 0 |
| peas and carrots, frozen | 3 oz | 81 | 187 | 45 | 8 | 0 |
| peas, blackeye, frozen | 3 oz | 6 | 388 | 109 | 19 | 0 |
| peas, whole, dried | ½ cup | 35 | 1005 | 340 | 60 | 1 |
| peas, split, dried | ½ cup | 40 | 895 | 348 | 63 | 1 |
| peas, split, cooked | 3 oz | 11 | 254 | 99 | 18 | 0.3 |
| peppers, green, raw | 1 large | 13 | 213 | 22 | 5 | 0.2 |
| peppers, green, cooked | 3 oz | 8 | 128 | 15 | 3 | 0.2 |
| pickles, cucumber, dill | 1 large | 1428 | 200 | 11 | 2 | 0.2 |
| pickles, cucumber, sour | 1 large | 1353 | | 10 | 2 | 0.2 |
| pickles, chow chow, sour | 1 large | 1338 | | 29 | 4 | 1 |
| pickles, relish, sweet | 3 oz | 610 | | 118 | 29 | 0.5 |
| pigeon peas, raw | ½ cup | 5 | 552 | 117 | 21 | 0.6 |
| potatoes, white, raw | 1 small | 3 | 407 | 76 | 17 | 0.1 |
| potatoes, white, no skin, baked | 1 small | 4 | 503 | 72 | 21 | 0.1 |

| CATEGORY & FOOD | PORTION | SODIUM (mg) | POTASSIUM (mg) | CALORIES | CARBOHYDRATES (g) | FAT (g) |
|---|---|---|---|---|---|---|
| potatoes, white, pared, boiled | 1 small | 2 | 285 | 65 | 15 | 0.1 |
| potatoes, white, boiled in skin | 1 med | 3 | 407 | 76 | 17 | 0.1 |
| potatoes, French fried | 10 | 3 | 427 | 137 | 18 | 7 |
| potatoes, hashed brown | ½ cup | 288 | 475 | 229 | 29 | 12 |
| potatoes, mashed | ½ cup | 331 | 250 | 94 | 12 | 4 |
| potatoes, French fried, frozen | 3 oz | 3 | 559 | 189 | 29 | 7 |
| prickly pears, raw | 3 oz | 2 | 142 | 36 | 9 | 0.1 |
| pumpkin, raw | 3 oz | 0.9 | 291 | 22 | 6 | 0.1 |
| pumpkin, canned | ½ cup | 2 | 276 | 38 | 8 | 0.3 |
| radish, red, raw | 10 small | 18 | 322 | 17 | 4 | 0.1 |
| rhubarb, raw | 3 oz | 2 | 215 | 14 | 3 | 0.1 |
| rhubarb, cooked with sugar | ½ cup | 3 | 271 | 188 | 48 | 0.1 |
| rhubarb, sweetened, frozen | ½ cup | 3 | 235 | 191 | 48 | 0.3 |
| rutabagas, raw | 3 oz | 4 | 205 | 39 | 9 | 0.1 |
| rutabagas, cubed, cooked | ½ cup | 4 | 167 | 35 | 8 | 0.1 |
| sauerkraut, canned | ½ cup | 560 | 105 | 14 | 3 | 0.2 |
| soybeans, raw | ½ cup | 5 | 1677 | 403 | 34 | 18 |
| soybeans, cooked | ½ cup | 2 | 540 | 130 | 11 | 6 |
| soybean curds | 3 oz | 6 | 36 | 62 | 2 | 4 |
| spinach, raw | 3 oz | 61 | 403 | 22 | 4 | 0.3 |
| spinach, cooked | ½ cup | 45 | 291 | 21 | 3 | 0.3 |

| | | | | | | |
|---|---|---|---|---|---|---|
| spinach, drained, canned | ½ cup | 212 | 227 | 22 | 3 | 0.5 |
| spinach, chopped, cooked, frozen | ½ cup | 52 | 333 | 23 | 4 | 0.3 |
| spinach, leaf, cooked, frozen | ½ cup | 49 | 362 | 24 | 4 | 0.3 |
| spinach, chopped, frozen | 3 oz | 40 | 306 | 18 | 3 | 0 |
| spinach, leaf, frozen | 3 oz | 64 | 379 | 18 | 3 | 0 |
| squash, summer, raw | ½ cup | 1 | 202 | 19 | 4 | 1 |
| squash, summer, cooked | ½ cup | 1 | 141 | 14 | 3 | 0.1 |
| squash, summer, cooked, frozen | ½ cup | 3 | 167 | 21 | 5 | 0.1 |
| squash, winter, raw | ½ cup | 1 | 369 | 50 | 12 | 0.3 |
| squash, winter, baked | ½ cup | 1 | 461 | 63 | 15 | 0.4 |
| squash, winter, cooked, frozen | ½ cup | 1 | 207 | 38 | 9 | 0.3 |
| squash, zucchini, frozen | 3 oz | 1 | 187 | 15 | 3 | 0 |
| sweet potatoes, raw | 1 small | 10 | 243 | 114 | 26 | 0.4 |
| sweet potatoes, baked in skin | 1 small | 12 | 300 | 141 | 33 | 0.5 |
| sweet potatoes, candied | 2 halves | 42 | 190 | 168 | 34 | 3 |
| sweet potatoes, canned | 1 small | 48 | 120 | 114 | 28 | 0.2 |
| tomatoes, green, raw | 1 small | 3 | 244 | 24 | 5 | 0.2 |
| tomatoes, ripe, raw | 1 small | 3 | 244 | 22 | 5 | 0.2 |
| tomatoes, cooked, boiled | ½ cup | 4 | 287 | 26 | 6 | 0.2 |
| tomatoes, canned | ½ cup | 130 | 217 | 21 | 4 | 0.2 |
| tomato catsup | 1 tbsp | 177 | 62 | 18 | 4 | 0.1 |
| tomato, chile sauce | 1 tbsp | 223 | 62 | 17 | 4 | 0.1 |
| tomato juice, canned | ½ cup | 200 | 227 | 19 | 4 | 0.1 |
| tomato paste, canned | 3 oz | 33 | 761 | 70 | 16 | 0.3 |

| CATEGORY & FOOD | PORTION | SODIUM (mg) | POTAS-SIUM (mg) | CALO-RIES | CARBO-HYDRATES (g) | FAT (g) |
|---|---|---|---|---|---|---|
| tomato puree, canned | ½ cup | 500 | 530 | 49 | 11 | 0.3 |
| turnip greens, canned | ½ cup | 236 | 243 | 18 | 3 | 0.3 |
| turnip greens, chopped, frozen | 3 oz | 10 | 158 | 18 | 2 | 0 |
| turnip, white root, diced, raw | ½ cup | 33 | 177 | 20 | 4 | 0.1 |
| turnip, white root, diced, cooked | ½ cup | 26 | 141 | 17 | 4 | 0.2 |
| water chestnuts, raw | 4 | 5 | 125 | 20 | 5 | 0.1 |
| watercress, raw | 10 sprigs | 5 | 28 | 2 | 0.3 | tr |
| **Vegetables—Canned, Especially Prepared for Low-Sodium Diets** | | | | | | |
| Asparagus, green—Balanced | 4 oz | 3 | | 16 | 3 | 0.1 |
| Asparagus, spears—Cellu | ½ cup | 5 | | 18 | 3 | 0 |
| Asparagus, cut spears—Featherweight | ½ cup | 5 | | 16 | 3 | 0 |
| Asparagus, green—S & W Nutradiet | ½ cup | 9 | | 17 | 3 | 0 |
| Asparagus—Tillie Lewis | ½ cup | <10 | | | | |
| Beans, green, cut—Arcadia | ½ cup | 10 | | 32 | 6 | 0 |
| Beans, green, cut—Balanced | 4 oz | 6 | | 24 | 4 | 0.1 |
| Beans, green, cut—Cellu | ½ cup | 0 | | 20 | 5 | 0 |
| Beans, green, cut—Featherweight | ½ cup | 0 | | 20 | 5 | 0 |
| Beans, green—S & W Nutradiet | ½ cup | 1 | | 20 | 9 | 0 |
| Beans, green—Tillie Lewis | ½ cup | <10 | | | | |
| Beans, wax, cut—Balanced | 4 oz | 2 | | 16 | 4 | 0.1 |

| | | | | | |
|---|---|---|---|---|---|
| Beans, wax, cut—Cellu | ½ cup | 0 | 20 | 5 | 0 |
| Beans, wax, cut—Featherweight | ½ cup | 0 | 20 | 5 | 0 |
| Beets, sliced—Arcadia | ½ cup | 57 | 51 | 11 | 0 |
| Beets, sliced—Balanced | 4 oz | 80 | 25 | 5 | 0.1 |
| Beets, sliced—Cellu | ½ cup | 55 | 40 | 10 | 0 |
| Beets, sliced—Featherweight | ½ cup | 55 | 40 | 10 | 0 |
| Beets, sliced—S & W Nutradiet | ½ cup | 40 | 35 | 9 | 0 |
| Beets, diced—Tillie Lewis | ½ cup | 75 | | | |
| Carrots, diced—Arcadia | ½ cup | 48 | 30 | 6 | 0 |
| Carrots, diced—Balanced | 4 oz | 40 | 28 | 6 | 0.2 |
| Carrots, diced—Tillie Lewis | ½ cup | 30 | 25 | 6 | 0 |
| Carrots, sliced—Cellu | ½ cup | 30 | 25 | 6 | 0 |
| Carrots, sliced—Featherweight | ½ cup | 50 | 30 | 7 | 0 |
| Carrots, sliced—S & W Nutradiet | ½ cup | 60 | | | |
| Corn—Tillie Lewis | ½ cup | <10 | | | |
| Corn, cream style—Featherweight | ½ cup | 5 | 80 | 18 | 1 |
| Corn, cream style—S & W Nutradiet | ½ cup | 4 | 100 | 21 | 1 |
| Corn, whole kernel—Arcadia | ½ cup | 3 | 95 | 19 | 0.5 |
| Corn, whole kernel—Balanced | 4 oz | 2 | 76 | 16 | 0.6 |
| Corn, whole kernel—Cellu | ½ cup | 15 | 65 | 15 | 0 |
| Corn, whole kernel—Featherweight | ½ cup | 10 | 70 | 16 | 1 |
| Corn, whole kernel—S & W Nutradiet | ½ cup | 9 | 40 | 8 | 0 |
| Lima beans—Arcadia | ½ cup | 5 | 135 | 25 | 0 |
| Lima beans—Balanced | 4 oz | 4 | 75 | 13 | 0.2 |

| CATEGORY & FOOD | PORTION | SODIUM (mg) | POTAS-SIUM (mg) | CALO-RIES | CARBO-HYDRATES (g) | FAT (g) |
|---|---|---|---|---|---|---|
| Lima beans, green—Cellu | ½ cup | 25 | | 73 | 16 | 0 |
| Lima beans, green—Featherweight | ½ cup | 25 | | 73 | 16 | 0 |
| Mushrooms, sliced—Balanced | 1 oz | 1 | | 5 | 0.9 | 0.1 |
| Peas, sweet—Arcadia | ½ cup | 9 | | 14 | 80 | 0 |
| Peas, sweet—Balanced | 4 oz | 2 | | 42 | 7 | 0.2 |
| Peas, sweet—Cellu | ½ cup | 5 | | 50 | 10 | 0 |
| Peas, sweet—Featherweight | ½ cup | 5 | | 50 | 10 | 0 |
| Peas, sweet—S & W Nutradiet | ½ cup | 9 | | 40 | 8 | 0 |
| Peas, sweet—Tillie Lewis | ½ cup | <10 | | | | |
| Peas and carrots—Arcadia | ½ cup | 24 | | 90 | 17 | 0.5 |
| Peas and carrots—Balanced | 4 oz | 16 | | 38 | 6 | 0.2 |
| Peas and carrots—S & W Nutradiet | ½ cup | 9 | | 35 | 7 | 0 |
| Spinach—Balanced | 4 oz | 8 | | 22 | 3 | 0.2 |
| Spinach—Cellu | ½ cup | 10 | | 26 | 3 | 0 |
| Spinach—Featherweight | ½ cup | 10 | | 26 | 3 | 0 |
| Tomatoes—Arcadia | ½ cup | 13 | | 25 | 6 | 0 |
| Tomatoes—Balanced | 4 oz | 3 | | 23 | 4 | 0.1 |
| Tomatoes—Cellu | ½ cup | 10 | | 20 | 4 | 0 |
| Tomatoes—Featherweight | ½ cup | 10 | | 20 | 4 | 0 |
| Tomatoes—Tillie Lewis | ½ cup | 15 | | | | |
| Tomatoes—stewed—Featherweight | ½ cup | 9 | | 35 | 9 | 0 |

| | | | | | | |
|---|---|---|---|---|---|---|
| Tomatoes, whole—S & W Nutradiet | ½ cup | 15 | | 25 | 5 | 0 |
| Tomato paste—Balanced | 4 oz | 35 | | 108 | 22 | 0.2 |
| Tomato paste—Cellu | ⅔ cup | 61 | | 150 | 35 | 0 |
| Vegetables, mixed—Featherweight | ½ cup | 20 | | 35 | 8 | 0 |
| **Vegetables—Juices** | | | | | | |
| tomato juice | 6 oz | 300 | 341 | 29 | 6 | |
| vegetable juice cocktail | 6 oz | 375 | 497 | 32 | 7 | 0.2 |
| **Vegetables—Juices Especially Prepared for Low-Sodium Diets** | | | | | | |
| Carrot juice—Arcadia | 6 oz | 200 | | 70 | 16 | 0 |
| Carrot juice—Hain | 6 oz | 18 | | 63 | 14 | 0 |
| Celery juice—Balanced | 6 oz | 229 | | 30 | 3 | 0.2 |
| Tomato juice—Arcadia | 6 oz | 20 | | 35 | 8 | 0 |
| Tomato juice—Featherweight | 6 oz | 5 | | 35 | 7 | 0 |
| Tomato juice—S & W Nutradiet | 6 oz | 10 | | 35 | 8 | 0 |
| Tomato juice—Tillie Lewis | 6 oz | 25 | | | | |
| Vegetable cocktail—S & W Nutradiet | 6 oz | 15 | | 35 | 8 | 0 |
| **Vegetables—Purees Especially Prepared for Low-Sodium Diets** | | | | | | |
| Puree of asparagus—Cellu | 1 cup | 10 | | 50 | 7 | 0 |
| Puree of green beans—Cellu | 1 cup | 10 | | 70 | 15 | 0 |

| CATEGORY & FOOD | PORTION | SODIUM (mg) | POTAS-SIUM (mg) | CALO-RIES | CARBO-HYDRATES (g) | FAT (g) |
|---|---|---|---|---|---|---|
| Puree of beets—Cellu | 1 cup | 120 | | 100 | 20 | 0 |
| Puree of carrots—Cellu | 1 cup | 60 | | 70 | 15 | 0 |
| Puree of peas—Cellu | 1 cup | 10 | | 140 | 29 | 0 |
| Puree of spinach—Cellu | 1 cup | 25 | | 45 | 7 | 0 |
| Puree of squash—Cellu | 1 cup | 10 | | 100 | 19 | 1 |
| Puree of tomato—Cellu | 1 cup | 10 | | 80 | 20 | 0 |

# List of Addresses

| BRAND NAME | WHERE TO WRITE TO (Manufacturer or Distributor) |
| --- | --- |
| Arcadia | Sherman Foods Inc., 276 Jackson Avenue, Bronx, N.Y. 10454. |
| Babara Bread Sticks | Babara Bakery, Inc., So. San Francisco, Calif. 94080. |
| Balanced | Balanced Foods Inc., 2500 83rd Street, North Bergen, N.J. |
| Bazzini's | A. L. Bazzini Co. Inc., 339 Greenwich Avenue, New York, N.Y. 10013. |
| Beatriz | Feder Trading Co., 351 Greenwich Avenue, New York, N.Y. 10013. |
| Bloomingdale's Bread | Bloomingdale's, 1000 Third Avenue, New York, N.Y. 10022. |
| Bread for Life | Breads for Life Bakery, Box 3484, Springfield, Mo. 65804. |
| | Cybros Inc., Box 851, Waukesha, Wisc. 53186. |
| | Hillsboro Bakery, Box 778, Hillsboro, Texas 76645. |
| | Life Line Foods, Rt 4, Pikeville, Tenn. 37367. |
| | Shiloah Farms, Sulphur Springs, Ark. 72768. |
| Campbell's | Campbell's Soup Company, Camden, N.J. 08101. |
| Capitol Charter | Capitol Charter Foods, Huntington, N.Y. 11743. |
| Cellu | Chicago Dietetic Supply, Inc., 405 East Shawmut, La Grange, Ill. 60525. |

| | |
|---|---|
| Chicken of the Sea | Ralston Purina Company, St. Louis, Mo. 63188. |
| Chico San | Sherman Foods Inc., 276 Jackson Avenue, Bronx, N.Y. 10454. |
| Daitch Shopwell Low-Salt Cottage Cheese | Daitch Shopwell, 400 Walnut Ave., Bronx, N.Y. 10454. |
| Devonsheer | Devonsheer Melba Corp., Devonsheer Building, Carlstadt, N.J. 07072. |
| Dutch Gouda | Otto Roth Cheese Distributor, 14 Empire Blvd., Moonachie, N.J. 07074. |
| D-Zerta | General Foods Consumer Center, 250 North Street, White Plains, N.Y. 10625. |
| El Molino | Sherman Foods Inc., 276 Jackson Avenue, Bronx, N.Y. 10454. |
| Estee | Estee Candy Company Inc., 169 Lackawanna Ave., Parsippany, N.J. 07054. |
| Featherweight | Chicago Dietetic Supply, Inc., 405 East Shawmut, La Grange, Ill. 60525. |
| Flavor Tree | Flavor Tree Foods Inc., 2645 N. Rose Street, Franklin Park, Ill. 60131. |
| Friendship Low-Salt Cottage Cheese | Friendship Food Products, 4900 Maspeth Ave., Maspeth, N.Y. 11378. |
| Goodman's | A. Goodman & Sons Inc., 21-07 41st Ave., Long Island City, N.Y. |
| Grielle | Jaret International Inc., 2670 Stillwell Ave., Brooklyn, N.Y. 11224. |
| Hain | Hain Pure Foods, 13660 South Figueroa St., Los Angeles, Calif. 90061. |
| Health Maid | Health Maid Natural Foods, Los Angeles, Calif. 90021. |
| Hol-Grain | Sherman Foods Inc., 276 Jackson Avenue, Bronx, N.Y. 10454. |
| Ka-Me | Sherman Foods Inc., 276 Jackson Avenue, Bronx, N.Y. 10454. |

| | |
|---|---|
| Keebler | Keebler Co. Inc., 75 State Street, Moonachie, N.J. |
| King Roland | American Roland Food Corp., 16 Hudson Street, New York, N.Y. 10013. |
| Levy's | Henry S. Levi & Son Inc., 95-115 Thamis Street, Brooklyn, N.Y. 11237. |
| Lilly Brand | Sherman Foods Inc., 276 Jackson Avenue, Bronx, N.Y. 10454. |
| Manischewitz | Manischewitz Food Products Inc., 340 Henderson St., Jersey City, N.J. |
| Morga | A & A, c/o Richter Brothers, 20 Capitol Drive, Moonachie, N.J. 07074. |
| Mother's | Mother's Food Products Inc., Avenue K North, Newark, N.J. |
| No-Cal | No-Cal Corp., College Point, N.Y. 11356. |
| Nu Vita | Nu Vita Foods Inc., 7524 S. W. Macadem Ave., Portland, Ore. 97219. |
| Pauly | Pauly Cheese Company, 1750 Morrow, Green Bay, Wisc. 54305. |
| Redwood Natural | Erewhon Natural and Organic Foods, 33 Farnsworth St., Boston, Mass. 02210, or 303 Howe Ave., Passaic, N.J. 07055. |
| Roland | American Roland Food Corp., 16 Hudson Street, New York, N.Y. 10013. |
| Sovex | Sovex Inc., P.O. Box Draw 310, Collegedale, Tenn. 37315. |
| Soy Town | Malt-O-Meal Company, Minneapolis, Minn. 55402. |
| Stella D'Oro | Stella D'Oro Biscuit Co., Inc., 184 West 237th St., Bronx, N.Y. |
| S & W Nutradiet | S & W Fine Foods (Address given by region)<br>(Central Pacific) 333 Schwerin St., San Francisco, Calif. 94134. |

| | |
|---|---|
| | (Chicago) 3350 N. Kedzie Ave., Chicago, Ill. 60618. |
| | (Los Angeles) 5010 Loma Vista Avenue, Los Angeles, Calif. 90051. |
| | (New York) 100 Caven Point Road, Jersey City, N.J. 07305. |
| | (Portland) 2233 N.W. 22nd Avenue, Portland, Ore. 97210. |
| | (St. Louis) 8838 Frost Avenue, Berkeley, Mo. 63134. |
| | (Utah/Idaho) 2040 East 33rd South, Salt Lake City, Utah, 84109. |
| | (Seattle) 2323 Airport Way, South, Seattle, Wash. 98134. |
| Tillie Lewis | Tillie Lewis Foods, Inc., Stockton, Calif. 95201. |
| Van Brode | Van Brode Milling Co., Inc., 56 Sterling Street, Clinton, Mass. 01510. |
| Van Winkle | Webster Van Winkle Corp., 5 Lafayette Ave., Summit, N.J. 07901. |
| Wuest | Wuest Diet Bakeries Inc., P.O. Box 7285, Jersey City, N.J. 07307. |

## ABOUT THE AUTHORS

J. PETER BRUNSWICK was born and educated in Europe and came to this country in 1946 after a career in journalism and photography. During World War II he served as a military correspondent and feature writer for the Royal Air Force. For the last twenty years he has been public relations counsel to an international airline. He has produced, written and directed several award-winning promotional films.

DOROTHY LOVE, New York drama critic award-winning producer, Broadway actress and mother of two daughters, is the wife of J. Peter Brunswick. She holds a teaching degree in mathematics. When it was discovered that Peter suffered from high blood pressure (hypertension), Ms. Love thoroughly researched hundreds of prepared food items available for the special low-sodium diet prescribed by Dr. Weinberg, in order to find ways of making it more interesting and palatable.

DR. ASSA WEINBERG received his medical degree from the University of Paris, France. He did research work in cellular biology at the Weizman Institute of Science, Rehovot, Israel, and New York University. He took his internship in Tel-Hashomer Hospital, Israel, and specialized in internal medicine in the United States where he finished his residency at Maimonides Medical Center, Brooklyn, New York. Dr. Weinberg is a known expert in acupuncture, the Chinese medicine, and he specializes in rheumatology.